Onychomycosis

Antonella Tosti • Tracey C. Vlahovic
Roberto Arenas
Editors

Onychomycosis

An Illustrated Guide to Diagnosis and Treatment

Springer

Editors
Antonella Tosti
Department of Dermatology &
Cutaneous Surgery
University of Miami
Miami, FL
USA

Roberto Arenas
Mycology Section
Dr. Manuel Gea González General Hospital
México, DF
México

Tracey C. Vlahovic
Department of Podiatric Medicine
Temple University School of Podiatric
Medicine
Philadelphia, PA
USA

ISBN 978-3-319-44852-7 ISBN 978-3-319-44853-4 (eBook)
DOI 10.1007/978-3-319-44853-4

Library of Congress Control Number: 2016963792

Printed on acid-free paper

This Springer imprint is published by Springer Nature
The registered company is Springer International Publishing AG
The registered company address is: Gewerbestrasse 11, 6330 Cham, Switzerland

Preface

Onychomycosis is the most common nail disorder that affects a very large number of patients worldwide. It is not just a cosmetic problem but an infection that requires treatment, and can cause important complications, particularly in patients with other commonly associated comorbidities such as diabetes or peripheral vascular diseases.

This book is designed as a very simple guide to help dermatologists, podiatrics, general practitioners, and nonmedical professionals to understand how onychomycosis develops, to diagnose it early, and select the best diagnostic test and treatment depending on clinical presentation and patient's characteristics. I have the pleasure to edit this book with two great friends and experts with special and unique skills in the field.

Dr. Tracey Vlahovic is Associate Professor at the Temple University School of Podiatric Medicine. She deals with onychomycosis daily and provides the very important podiatric knowledge and expertise. Dr. Roberto Arenas is an internationally recognized opinion leader in mycology, and his contribution is very important to define gold standards for diagnosis and treatment of onychomycosis. I hope you will enjoy this book and utilize the information for the best quality of care of your patients.

Miami, FL, USA — Antonella Tosti, MD

Contents

Contributors

Jennifer L. Abrahams, MD Department of Dermatology and Cutaneous Surgery, University of Miami Miller School of Medicine, Miami, FL, USA

Chris G. Adigun, MD Board Certified Dermatologist and Nail Specialist, Chapel Hill, NC, USA

Roberto Arenas, MD Mycology Section, Dr. Manuel Gea González General Hospital, México, DF, México

Daniel Asz-Sigall, MD Mycology Section, Dr. Manuel Gea González General Hospital, México, DF, México

Christina Bui, BA Department of Podiatric Medicine, Temple University School of Podiatric Medicine, Philadelphia, PA, USA

Cara L. Dawes, DPM Department of Podiatry, Chestnut Hill Hospital, Philadelphia, PA, USA

Ramón Fernández-Martínez, MD Mycology Section, Dr. Manuel Gea González General Hospital, México, DF, México

Paola Flores-Gavilán, MD Dermatology Division, Dermatopathology Section, Dr. Manuel Gea González General Hospital, México, DF, México

Emilie Fowler, BS University of Miami Miller School of Medicine, Department of Dermatology and Cutaneous Surgery, Miami, FL, USA

Jeremy Brandon Freedman, BA University of Miami Miller School of Medicine, Miami, FL, USA

George Glinos, BS University of Miami Miller School of Medicine, Miami, FL, USA

Rigoberto Hernández-Castro, MSc, PhD Department of Ecology of Pathogens Agents, Dr. Manuel Gea González General Hospital, México, DF, México

Audrey A. Jacobsen, BA Department of Dermatology and Cutaneous Surgery, University of Miami Miller School of Medicine, Miami, FL, USA

Miriam America Jesus-Silva, M.Sc, MD Clínica de Onco-Dermatología, Facultad de Medicina. UNAM, Universidad Nacional Autónoma de México, Mexico, Mexico

Pablo Campo-Macias, MD Dermatology, Aranda de la Parra, León, Guanajuato, Mexico

Austin J. Maddy, BA Department of Dermatology and Cutaneous Surgery, University of Miami Miller School of Medicine, Miami, FL, USA

Stephanie Mlacker, BS Department of Dermatology and Cutaneous Surgery, University of Miami Miller School of Medicine, Miami, FL, USA

Gabriela Moreno-Coutiño, MD Mycology Section, Dr. Manuel Gea González General Hospital, México, DF, México

Rodrigo Roldan-Marin, MD Faculty of Medicine, Universidad Nacional Autonoma de Mexico, Circuito Escolar s/n, Anexo 1 Facultad de Medicine, Ciudad Universitaria, Entre Div. Gral CCH and Services Medicos VI, Mexico, Mexico

Julieta Ruiz-Esmenjaud, MD Mycology Section, Dr. Manuel Gea González General Hospital, México, DF, México

Joshua A. Sebag, BA Department of Podiatric Medicine, Temple University School of Podiatric Medicine, Philadelphia, PA, USA

Vidhi V. Shah, BA Department of Dermatology and Cutaneous Surgery, University of Miami Miller School of Medicine, Miami, FL, USA

Kyle Shaw, BS Department of Podiatric Medicine, Temple University School of Podiatric Medicine, Philadelphia, PA, USA

Edoardo Torres-Guerrero, MD Mycology Section, Dr. Manuel Gea González General Hospital, México, DF, México

Antonella Tosti, MD Department of Dermatology and Cutaneous Surgery, University of Miami Miller School of Medicine, Miami, FL, USA

Sonia Toussaint-Caire, MD Dermatology Division, Dermatopathology Section, Dr. Manuel Gea González General Hospital, México, DF, México

Diana C. Vega, MD Mycology Section, Dr. Manuel Gea González General Hospital, México, DF, México

Joseph Vella, DPM Impression Foot and Ankle, Gilbert, AZ, USA

Tracey C. Vlahovic, DPM, FFPM RCPS (Glasg) Department of Podiatric Medicine, Temple University School of Podiatric Medicine, Philadelphia, PA, USA

Part I
Is Onychomycosis a Disease or a Cosmetic Problem?

Chapter 1
Fungi and the Nails

Jeremy Brandon Freedman and Antonella Tosti

Key Features

- Fungal nail infections are incredibly common.
- The most common fungal pathogens of the nails are dermatophytes, but non-dermatophytic molds and yeasts can be implicated as well.
- Both the fungal species and their mechanism of invasion are major determinants of clinical presentation.
- The most common pattern of fungal invasion is distal lateral subungual onychomycosis (DLSO).
- Keratin invasion is an important part of initiating and establishing a fungal nail infection. Unfortunately, the exact mechanisms are still not fully understood.

Introduction

From a clinical perspective, nails are simply specialized keratin structures on the dorsal surfaces of our fingers and toes. To the average person, however, they represent so much more. Nails are protective, useful for grasping fine objects, perfect for scratching itches, and important to an individual's overall appearance: people spend time cutting, filing, and sometimes decorating them in order to look "presentable." Understanding that, it's easy to see how diseases of the nail can have substantial physical and psychosocial consequences [1].

J.B. Freedman, BA • A. Tosti, MD (✉)
Department of Dermatology and Cutaneous Surgery,
University of Miami, Miami, FL 33136, USA
e-mail: JBFreedman@miami.edu; atosti@med.miami.edu

A. Tosti et al. (eds.), *Onychomycosis*, DOI 10.1007/978-3-319-44853-4_1

Indeed, individuals with nail dystrophies often suffer from considerable pain and discomfort, can have difficulty walking, and are at risk for significant complications, including bacterial superinfection and cellulitis [2]. Moreover, recent studies have shown that those afflicted with certain nail dystrophies are often shunned in their personal and professional lives due to the unsightly disfigurement [3].

Although there are a variety of disorders (both cutaneous and systemic) that can affect the nails, more than half of all nail dystrophies are caused by fungal infections (onychomycosis) [4]. Unfortunately, fungal nail infections are often difficult to definitively diagnose, as many nail disorders (fungal and non-fungal alike) have the potential to cause a wide variety of nail abnormalities. Consequently, any given abnormality may be the manifestation of various diseases. Therefore, it's important that any clinical suspicion of onychomycosis be confirmed with laboratory testing. Additionally, there are many species of fungi that can invade the nails and multiple mechanisms of fungal invasion, both of which can contribute to the clinical presentation [5, 6].

While fungal infections of the nail are normally superficial and very rarely life threatening, many are particularly difficult to treat, and patients are often left either entirely without treatment or with incompletely cured infections and recurrences.

Since practically every patient who visits a physician's office has nails, and the prevalence of onychomycosis can climb as high as 50 % in patients over 70 years of age [7], it is extremely likely that most physicians will encounter many cases of fungal nail infections during their years of practice. It makes sense, therefore, for every physician to have a good understanding of how fungus can affect the nails.

State of Art

As mentioned, onychomycosis can be caused by different species of fungi, specifically dermatophytes, non-dermatophytic molds, and yeasts [8].

The vast majority of fungal nail infections are caused by dermatophytes (parasitic fungal organisms that feed on keratin) [9], particularly *Trichophyton rubrum* and *Trichophyton mentagrophytes*. Overall, those species are responsible for 80–90 % of all fungal nail infections [10].

Other fungal pathogens that affect the nails are non-dermatophytic molds (NDMs), the five most frequently isolated organisms of which are *Scopulariopsis brevicaulis*, *Fusarium* species, *Aspergillus* species, *Scytalidium dimidiatum*, and *Acremonium* species [5, 11]. These infections often respond poorly to antifungal therapy and are difficult to cure [5]. Thankfully, they are relatively uncommon, with an estimated prevalence of approximately 10 % [11]. Their clinical presentation is very similar to that of dermatophyte onychomycosis, but in addition is typically associated with marked periungual inflammation and possible purulent discharge [5, 11, 12].

Rarely, onychomycosis can be caused by yeasts [13]. *Candida* onychomycosis is more common in fingernails, and generally occurs only in patients who are

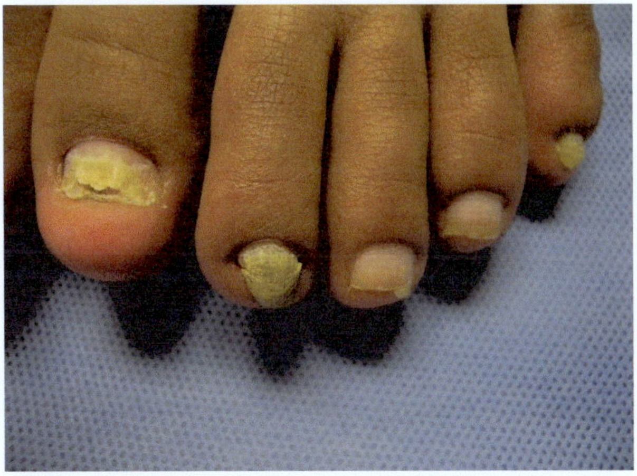

Fig. 1.1 Candida onychomycosis in a patient with chronic mucocutaneous candidiasis

immunosuppressed [12], particularly those with chronic mucocutaneous candidiasis (Fig. 1.1). Note that *Candida* is a component of the normal flora in humans, as well as a commensal of the skin, and commonly colonizes the underside of the nail without causing pathological effects [4, 6].

Aside from the multiple fungal culprits, there are also multiple routes of invasion that fungi can use to infect the nail. However, in order to properly understand the different mechanisms of fungal invasion, it's important to first have a solid grasp of nail anatomy and the process of nail growth.

The nail consists of the nail matrix, the nail plate, the underlying nail bed, and the nail folds. The nail plate is composed of hard, keratinized cells which grow out of the nail matrix – the distal, visible part of which looks like a half-moon and is called the lunula – and emerges from beneath the proximal nail fold and cuticle (which protects the nail matrix from the environment), bordered on either side by the lateral nail folds. It extends along the nail bed, and is normally cut distally, just past the hyponychium (where the skin of the fingertip meets the nail bed), at the free edge of the nail (Fig. 1.2) [14, 15].

There are five generally accepted patterns of fungal nail infections, each utilizing a slightly different mechanism of invasion. They are: distal lateral subungual onychomycosis (DLSO), superficial onychomycosis (SO), proximal subungual onychomycosis (PSO), endonyx onychomycosis (EO), and total dystrophic onychomycosis (TDO) [16].

The most common form of fungal invasion of the nail is DLSO [4, 6]. This occurs when fungus invades the nail bed and undersurface of the nail plate via the hyponychium (usually as an extension of tinea pedis/manuum), and spreads proximally along the longitudinally oriented rete ridges of the nail bed.

SO was previously known as superficial white onychomycosis (SWO), but that term became too narrow once SO was found to present with other features (such as deep penetration, brown/black pigmentation, etc.) depending on the organism involved [6]. SO occurs when the fungus localizes superficially on the dorsal nail

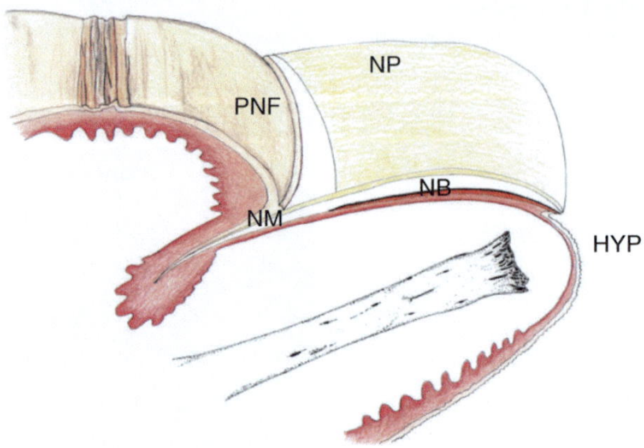

Fig. 1.2 This illustration of a sagittal section of the finger provides us with a visual of some internal and external details of nail anatomy. The nail plate (*NP*) grows out of the nail matrix (*NM*) and extends along the nail bed (*NB*). It is bordered proximally by the proximal nail fold (*PNF*) and distally by the hyponychium (*HYP*)

plate and forms colonies (seen as opaque, scaly plaques with distinct edges) that are easily scraped away. Some NDMs actually penetrate deeper into the nail plate, causing a deep, diffuse SO that can extend past the proximal nail fold and is visible through the cuticle [5, 17].

In PSO, the fungal elements invade the deeper, ventral aspect of the nail plate from the proximal portion of the nail and migrate distally, causing a patch or a band of leukonychia that moves distally with nail growth. PSO is a relatively uncommon subtype that can suggest the possibility of HIV infection or other types of immunosuppression [4]. It can also occur secondarily to paronychia (infection and inflammation of the nail folds) [6]. As mentioned above, when PSO is associated with periungual inflammation, we should suspect a mold infection.

EO occurs when the fungus invades the distal nail plate directly, without any involvement of the nail bed. This is a very rare presentation, characterized by nail plate invasion without subungual hyperkeratosis (because the nail bed is spared) [6, 16].

Besides those five general classifications, there are some patients that present with features from multiple forms of nail infection, called mixed pattern onychomycosis (MPO) [6, 16]. The two most common examples of this are when a nail affected with DLSO develops SO as well (especially in an area where another toe overrides it) and when SO extends under the proximal nail fold, creating an increased risk of PSO.

Eventually, if the fungal infections are allowed to progress, the entire nail will become thick and dystrophic. This end-stage nail disease is referred to as total dystrophic onychomycosis (TDO) (Fig. 1.3) [4, 6, 16].

Before any of these classical presentations can occur, however, the fungus must first initiate and establish an infection. In order for it to do that, it needs to accomplish three steps: make contact, adhere to the stratum corneum, and invade the keratin layers [18]. We will examine how dermatophytes accomplish these steps.

The first phase occurs when an individual comes into contact with a contaminated surface or another affected individual. Naturally, certain areas of the body are more susceptible to infection than others, owing to anatomic and/or environmental

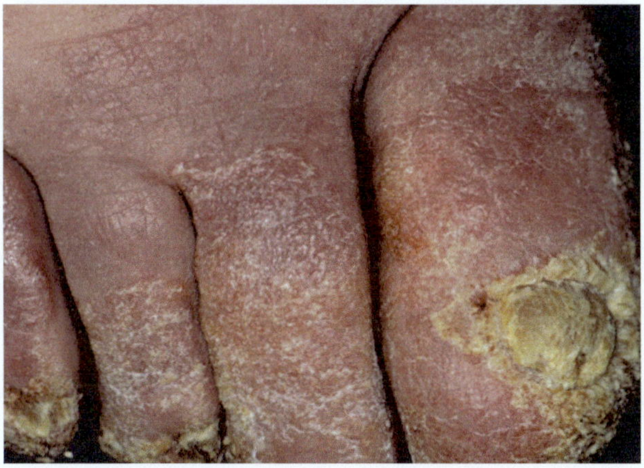

Fig. 1.3 Total dystrophic onychomycosis. Note the severe concomitant tinea pedis

factors such as humidity, temperature, pH, etc. Understanding this helps to explain the greatly increased frequency of toenail compared to fingernail onychomycosis (a ratio of 19:1) [19]. The warm, moist, confined environment provided by our occlusive footwear, combined with slower toenail than fingernail growth and less blood flow to the area, all combine to make the feet and toes specifically vulnerable. There are also patients with a general predisposition to contracting onychomycosis due to genetic factors [20–22].

After contact is made, the fungal arthroconidia (a primitive spore type, formed by fragmentation or disarticulation of existing hyphae) spend the next few hours (between 2 and 12) completing the second phase: adhering to the outer layer of the skin [18, 23]. Regrettably, little is known about the specific factors that mediate dermatophyte adherence [23]. We know the fungal arthroconidia produce both short and long adhesive fibrils that anchor them to the tissue surface and that the fungus secretes proteases that may modify both the surface of the epithelial cells and the fungus itself, inducing conformational changes that potentially facilitate adherence [18, 23, 24]. We also know dermatophytes express certain adhesins specific for carbohydrates present on the skin surface – but these have not been sufficiently investigated for us to determine what, if any, role they play in adherence [18, 23].

It's important to note the resilience of the arthroconidia, as they are often the primary form involved in the spread of infection. Since they have thicker cell walls and no immediate exogenous nutritional requirements, they can persist in the environment, even under what would otherwise be hostile conditions [25, 26]. Additionally, fungal spores are greatly resistant to antifungal medication, requiring a dose 10–1000 times higher than that necessary to kill growing hyphae cells [25, 27]. This is one of the contributing factors to the high recurrence rate of onychomycosis: treatment often fails to eradicate the resistant arthroconidia, and a reservoir of infection is left behind [25, 28].

Once the dermatophytes have adhered to the stratum corneum, they release enzymes (keratinases, lipases, nonspecific proteases, etc.) which have their optimal activity at the pH level of the human skin [29]. This begins the third and final phase, by helping the germinating arthroconidia's fungal hyphae penetrate the host tissue and scavenge for nutrients, digesting keratin into shorter peptides and amino acids to be assimilated [23, 29]. However, much of the process of fungal invasion, like the process of fungal adherence, is still not fully understood [23].

Unfortunately, the value of animal models in helping us understand dermatophyte infections is limited, as they do not perfectly mirror human infections [30]. Furthermore, most human dermatophyte infections are caused by *T. rubrum*, which specifically requires a human host. Animal models can still be useful, though, for evaluating diagnostic procedures and testing new treatments [30].

Outlook: Future Developments

Treating onychomycosis is problematic for a variety of reasons. Oral therapy is more effective than topical therapy, but it's expensive, requires monitoring for toxicity, and can result in multiple drug interactions. Topical therapy is a long process that often requires nail debridement and multiple return visits and still delivers a relatively poor success rate. The very nature of the hard, protective nail plate itself makes it difficult for topical drugs to reach the fungal pathogens beneath it.

Thankfully, recent studies have offered insights that may improve our topical treatment options. For example, a new study has definitively shown that structural changes which occur during fungal infections cause the nail plate to become more permeable to small, hydrophilic molecules [31]. This is important information, as currently, most topical drugs are delivered in a relatively lipophilic substrate and do not take full advantage of the increased permeability.

Additionally, although the process of dermatophyte fungal infection (specifically adhesion and invasion) might not yet be fully understood, studies are currently underway in an effort to analyze the dermatophyte genome and their gene expression profile during infection in order to build a basis for the development of new drugs for treatment and prevention [23].

Summary for the Clinician

Onychomycosis is a very common infection that can be caused by a variety of fungal species. The vast majority of cases are caused by dermatophytes, but non-dermatophytic molds and yeasts can be implicated as well.

Fungi can invade the nail using multiple mechanisms, and that will affect the clinical presentation of the disease. It's important to properly distinguish between the different types, as treatment differs depending on the fungal species and mechanism of invasion.

Research is ongoing into the exact mechanisms of fungal adhesion and invasion. Hopefully, those discoveries will lead to improved treatments.

Clinical Pearls

- Since onychomycosis can be caused by multiple species of fungi, it is important to confirm the causative agent with laboratory techniques.

References

1. Chacon A, Franca K, Fernandez A, Nouri K. Psychosocial impact of onychomycosis: a review. Int J Dermatol. 2013;52(11):1300–7.
2. Reich A, Szepietowski JC. Health-related quality of life in patients with nail disorders. Am J Clin Dermatol. 2011;12(5):313–20.
3. Chan HH, Wong ET, Yeung CK. Psychosocial perception of adults with onychomycosis: a blinded, controlled comparison of 1,017 adult Hong Kong residents with or without onychomycosis. Biopsychosoc Med. 2014;8:15.
4. Piraccini BM, Alessandrini A. Onychomycosis: a review. J Fungi. 2015;1:30–43.
5. Tosti A, Piraccini BM, Lorenzi S. Onychomycosis caused by nondermatophytic molds: clinical features and response to treatment of 59 cases. J Am Acad Dermatol. 2000;42(2 Pt 1):217–24.
6. Hay RJ, Baran R. Onychomycosis: a proposed revision of the clinical classification. J Am Acad Dermatol. 2011;65(6):1219–27.
7. Thomas J, Jacobson GA, Narkowicz CK. Toenail onychomycosis: an important global disease burden. J Clin Pharm Ther. 2010;35(5):497–519.
8. Elewski BE. Onychomycosis: pathogenesis, diagnosis, and management. Clin Microbiol Rev. 1998;11(3):415–29.
9. Foster KW, Ghannoum MA, Elewski BE. Epidemiologic surveillance of cutaneous fungal infection in the United States from 1999 to 2002. J Am Acad Dermatol. 2004;50(5):748–52.
10. Loo DS. Onychomycosis in the elderly: drug treatment options. Drugs Aging. 2007;24(4):293–302.
11. Gupta AK, Drummond-Main C, Cooper EA, et al. Systematic review of nondermatophyte mold onychomycosis: diagnosis, clinical types, epidemiology, and treatment. J Am Acad Dermatol. 2012;66(3):494–502.
12. Tosti A, Piraccini BM, Lorenzi S, et al. Treatment of nondermatophyte mold and Candida onychomycosis. Dermatol Clin. 2003;21(3):491–7. vii.
13. Ebihara M, Makimura K, Sato K, et al. Molecular detection of dermatophytes and nondermatophytes in onychomycosis by nested polymerase chain reaction based on 28S ribosomal RNA gene sequences. Br J Dermatol. 2009;161(5):1038–44.
14. Haneke E. Surgical anatomy of the nail apparatus. Dermatol Clin. 2006;24(3):291–6.
15. Cohen JL, Scher RK, Pappert AS. The nail and fungus infections. In: Elewski B, editor. Cutaneous fungal infections. New York: Igaku-Shoin Inc.; 1992. p. 106–22.
16. Baran R, Hay RJ, Tosti A, et al. A new classification of onychomycosis. Br J Dermatol. 1998;139(4):567–71.
17. Piraccini BM, Tosti A. White superficial onychomycosis: epidemiological, clinical, and pathological study of 79 patients. Arch Dermatol. 2004;140(6):696–701.
18. Mendez-Tovar LJ. Pathogenesis of dermatophytosis and tinea versicolor. Clin Dermatol. 2010;28(2):185–9.
19. Gupta AK, Jain HC, Lynde CW, et al. Prevalence and epidemiology of onychomycosis in patients visiting physicians' offices: a multicenter Canadian survey of 15,000 patients. J Am Acad Dermatol. 2000;43(2 Pt 1):244–8.
20. Zaias N, Tosti A, Rebell G, et al. Autosomal dominant pattern of distal subungual onychomycosis caused by Trichophyton rubrum. J Am Acad Dermatol. 1996;34(2 Pt 1):302–4.

21. Zaias N, Rebell G. Chronic dermatophytosis syndrome due to Trichophyton rubrum. Int J Dermatol. 1996;35(9):614–7.
22. Gupta AK, Simpson FC, Brintnell WC. Do genetic mutations and genotypes contribute to onychomycosis? Dermatology. 2014;228(3):207–10.
23. Baldo A, Monod M, Mathy A, et al. Mechanisms of skin adherence and invasion by dermatophytes. Mycoses. 2012;55(3):218–23.
24. Hay RJ. Fungal skin infections. Arch Dis Child. 1992;67(9):1065–7.
25. Hashimoto T, Blumenthal HJ. Survival and resistance of Trichophyton mentagrophytes arthrospores. Appl Environ Microbiol. 1978;35(2):274–7.
26. Yazdanparast SA, Barton RC. Arthroconidia production in Trichophyton rubrum and a new ex vivo model of onychomycosis. J Med Microbiol. 2006;55(Pt 11):1577–81.
27. Seidl HP, Jäckel A, Müller J, et al. Sporicidal effect of amorolfine and other antimycotics used in the therapy of fungal nail infections. Mycoses. 2015;58(10):610–9.
28. Ghannoum M, Isham N. Fungal nail infections (onychomycosis): a never-ending story? PLoS Pathog. 2014;10(6):e1004105.
29. Martinez-Rossi NM, Persinoti GF, Peres NT, et al. Role of pH in the pathogenesis of dermatophytoses. Mycoses. 2012;55(5):381–7.
30. Saunte DM, Hasselby JP, Brillowska-Dabrowska A, et al. Experimental guinea pig model of dermatophytosis: a simple and useful tool for the evaluation of new diagnostics and antifungals. Med Mycol. 2008;46(4):303–13.
31. McAuley WJ, Jones SA, Traynor MJ, et al. An investigation of how fungal infection influences drug penetration through onychomycosis patient's nail plates. Eur J Pharm Biopharm. 2016;102:178–84.

Chapter 2
Predisposing Factors for Onychomycosis

Audrey A. Jacobsen and Antonella Tosti

Key Features

- Onychomycosis is the most prevalent nail disease with a significant burden on quality of life.
- Age is the principal non-modifiable risk factor for onychomycosis development.
- Medical conditions such as diabetes, HIV infection, immunosuppressed states, concurrent tinea pedis, and peripheral artery disease increase the risk for onychomycosis.
- Physical and environmental factors that increase risk include obesity, certain athletic activities, and possibly smoking.

Introduction

Onychomycosis is the most prevalent nail disease, representing up to 50 % of all nail problems and 30 % of all dermatophytoses [1]. It is estimated that over 10 million individuals suffer from onychomycosis in the United States [2], affecting between 2 and 26 % of the general population [2–6]. In Europe, tinea pedis and onychomycosis are estimated to affect a quarter of individuals [7]. Onychomycosis causes a significant burden on quality of life, causing high rates of embarrassment and other psychological sequelae [8–10], in addition to physical costs including pain and loss of dexterity [11].

A.A. Jacobsen, BA • A. Tosti, MD (✉)
Department of Dermatology and Cutaneous Surgery,
University of Miami, Miami, FL 33136, USA
e-mail: ajacobsen@miami.edu; atosti@med.miami.edu

A. Tosti et al. (eds.), *Onychomycosis*, DOI 10.1007/978-3-319-44853-4_2

Onychomycosis is caused most commonly by dermatophytes followed by yeasts, then non-dermatophytic molds [12]. The predisposing factors, as well as the factors for relapse and reinfection, are important for clinicians to understand to optimize management strategies for at-risk individuals. Predisposing factors include genetic and non-modifiable risk factors, medical conditions, and physical and environmental influences (Table 2.1).

State of Art

Genetic and Non-modifiable Risk Factors

Age is the principal non-modifiable risk factor for the development of onychomycosis. The prevalence of onychomycosis increases significantly with age [13].

Estimates range from 15 to 47.7 % [8, 14, 15] in the elderly, compared to 0.44–0.6 % [8, 16] of children and 10–20 % [8] of adults. Poor peripheral circulation, repetitive nail trauma, diminished immune response, slower nail growth, and duration of exposure to fungi have been suggested as reasons for this age disparity [8]. However, while children experience the lowest prevalence, it is more often

Clinical Pearls (Table 2.1)

Table 2.1 Predisposing factors for onychomycosis

Category	Factors cited in the literature
Genetic and non-modifiable risk factors	Older age [8, 13–15] Male sex [13] Parent or child with onychomycosis [13] Autosomal dominant pattern of inheritance in distal subungual onychomycosis [18–21]. HLA-DR53 [22] and HLA-DR6 [23] may confer protection ICAM-1 deficiency in chronic nail candidiasis [25] Single nucleotide polymorphism in the Dectin-1 gene [26]
Medical conditions	Diabetes [27–31] Immunosuppression [13, 18, 33, 35] HIV infection [18, 33, 34] Concurrent tinea pedis infection [13, 36] Psoriasis [13, 37, 38] Peripheral arterial disease [40–42] Venous insufficiency [41, 43]
Physical and environmental factors	Athletic activity, especially swimming [2, 13, 44, 45] Nail trauma [8] Obesity [8, 46] Smoking [40] Increased prevalence of opportunistic fungal pathogens in the environment [47]

misdiagnosed in them [2]. Lastly, gender also plays a role; most studies have found a higher prevalence in males [13].

Genetic factors, such as inheritance patterns, the role of human leukocyte antigens (HLA), and intensity of immune response [17], have also been studied as potential predisposing factors. Distal subungual onychomycosis caused by *T. rubrum* shows an autosomal dominant pattern of inheritance (Fig. 2.1) [18–21]. Having a parent or child with onychomycosis has also been shown to be a predisposing factor [13].

Several studies have identified a possible role of HLA in the immune response of T cells to fungal peptides; HLA-DR53 [22] and HLA-DR6 [23] may confer protection. However, studies of the role of HLA are inconsistent as another study suggested HLA-controlled immunity is unlikely [24]. Other genetic risk factors may include ICAM-1 deficiency in familial chronic nail candidiasis [25]. Additionally, an allele of the Dectin-1 gene with a single nucleotide polymorphism was identified in a family with a propensity for onychomycosis and vulvovaginal candidiasis [26].

Medical Factors

Acquired medical conditions are significant predisposing factors for onychomycosis. Comorbid cutaneous, vascular, endocrine, infectious, and oncologic conditions have all been implicated [8]. For example, diabetics have a significantly higher

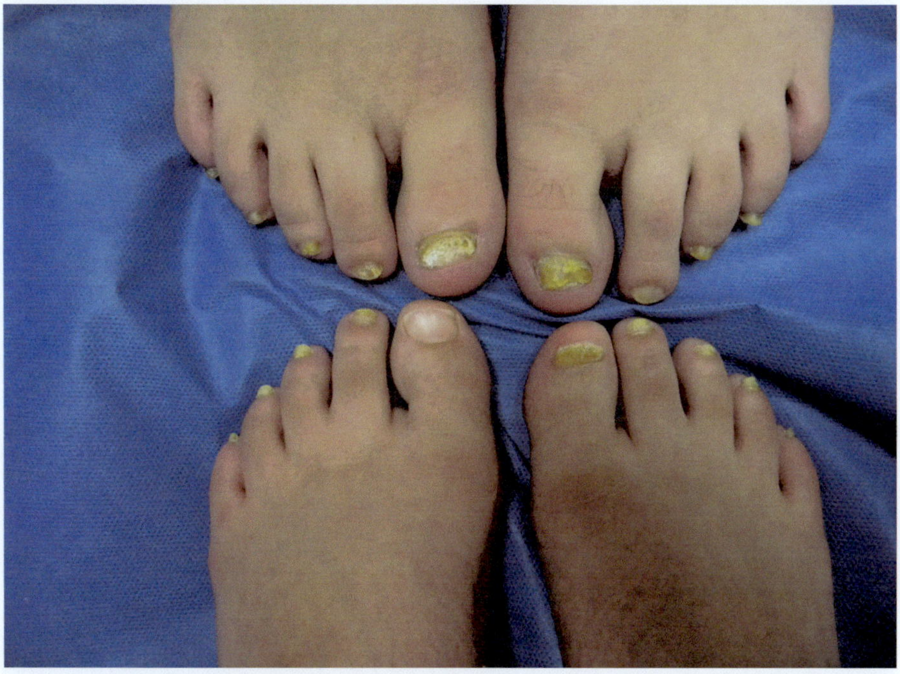

Fig. 2.1 Distal lateral subungual onychomycosis due to T. rubrum in two sisters

likelihood of developing onychomycosis [27, 28], with an estimated one third of diabetics affected (Fig. 2.2) [27, 29]. In patients with diabetic foot complications, the prevalence is even higher, with 53.3 % of patients affected in one study [30]. Additionally, onychomycosis in diabetics can lead to serious complications including limb-threatening infections due to the micro- and macrovascular and neurologic sequelae of diabetes [29]. Diabetics are also prone to less common fungal organisms including Aspergillus [31]. Lastly, there is some evidence that onychomycosis in diabetics may be resistant to treatment, but studies are conflicting [8, 32].

Immunosuppressed patients such as those with HIV [18, 33] or cancer [13] are also at increased risk of developing onychomycosis. Studies of HIV-infected individuals have estimated a prevalence of a quarter [33] to 30.3% [18, 34] compared to 6.9 [33] to 12.6 % [34] of immunocompetent controls (Fig. 2.3). Associated factors in HIV-positive individuals include a CD4 count of 370 or less, family history, history of tinea pedis, use of swimming pools, and walking barefoot [33]. Proximal subungual onychomycosis is also more prevalent in immunosuppressed patients [33, 35]. Recurrent proximal subungual onychomycosis was identified in a patient with a defect in defect of polymorphonuclear chemotaxis [35]. There is also a risk of systemic dissemination in immunocompromised patients, particularly of Fusarium species [18]. Importantly, in patients with a compromised immune system, the usual dose and treatment length may not be appropriate and drug interactions may be an issue [18].

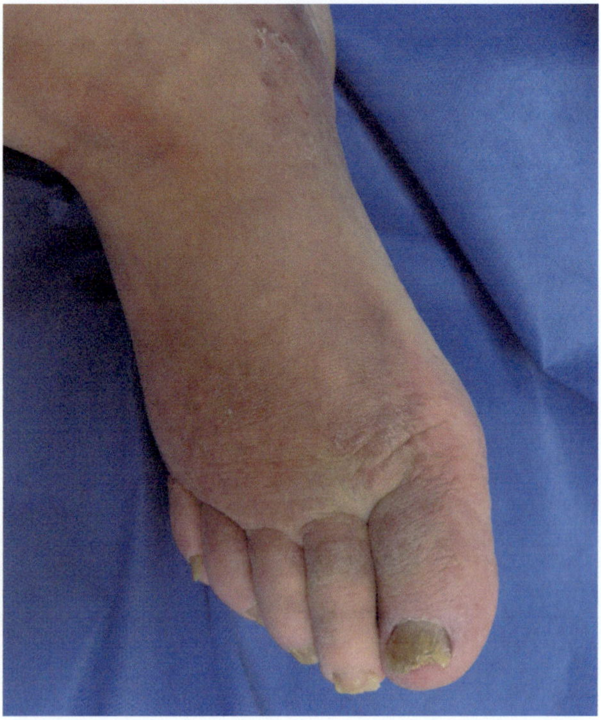

Fig. 2.2 Distal lateral subungual onychomycosis and tinea pedis in a diabetic patient

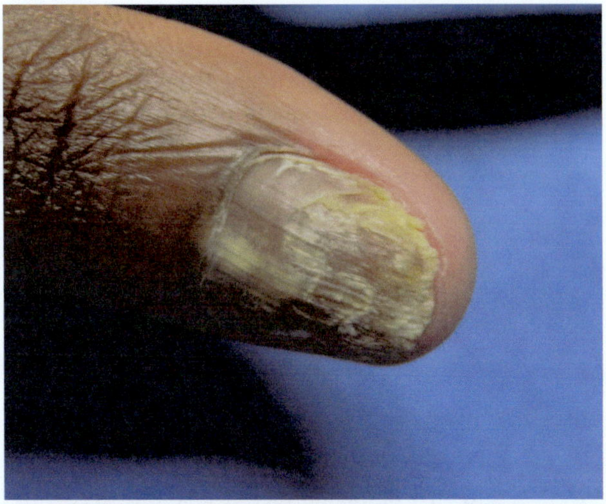

Fig. 2.3 Proximal subungual onychomycosis in a patient with HIV infection

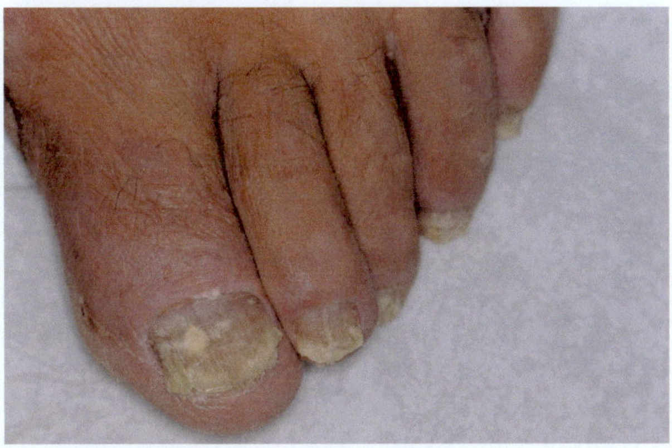

Fig. 2.4 Distal lateral subungual onychomycosis and psoriasis

Concurrent tinea pedis infection increases the risk of onychomycosis [13, 36]. Both the moccasin and interdigitalis form are implicated [13]. Tinea pedis is also associated with subclinical onychomycosis in which fungal organisms are isolated from the nails without any clinical manifestations. In a study of 35 patients with tinea pedis, 6 cases (17 %) had subclinical onychomycosis compared to 1 case (1.5 %) in the 66 control subjects [36]. Subclinical onychomycosis is also common in diabetics and is associated with neuropathy and poor glycemic control [29].

Dermatophytic invasion of involved psoriatic nails is more common than previously thought (Fig. 2.4) [37]. The organisms isolated from patients with psoriasis are similar to those of the normal population, although the odds of having onychomycosis are greater than those of the same age and sex [13, 38]. However, in an in-patient setting, the prevalence of onychomycosis among patients with psoriasis may not be different from those with other skin disorders [39].

Peripheral arterial disease and venous insufficiency are also thought to confer a greater risk for onychomycosis [40–42]. However, studies are conflicting. Ozkan et al. found a significant increase in onychomycosis in patients with venous insufficiency but not in peripheral arterial disease [41]. This contrasts with a study by Fukunaga et al. who found a significantly higher proportion of onychomycosis in patients with peripheral arterial disease than those without [43].

Other medical conditions that may show an increased risk include angioedema, urticaria, and asthma [13]. However, these connections were not strong and are not confirmed by any additional studies.

Physical and Environmental Risk Factors

Physical and environmental factors also play a role in the development of onychomycosis. For example, frequent athletic activity appears to increase the risk of onychomycosis [2, 44]. Athletes are more susceptible to developing toenail problems in general and onychomycosis is a common observance. However, the association between activity level and development onychomycosis is stronger in children and young adults than in older adults [2]. Swimming in particular has been associated with higher risk in several studies [13]; one study estimated the risk for toenail onychomycosis was three times higher for swimmers than the general population [45]. Further, wearing airtight shoes for sports like running and cycling is often associated with onychomycosis [2, 8].

Other physical and environmental factors that may increase the risk of onychomycosis include obesity [8, 46], nail damage [8], smoking [40], and prevalence of opportunistic fungal pathogens in a given environment [47]. Obesity may also negatively affect treatment outcomes; in two studies, topical 10 % efinaconazole was less effective in overweight or obese patients [8]. The evidence for smoking is less clear as studies are conflicting. One study found no correlation, but had too few heavy smokers to make any significant conclusions [13]. Another study by Gupta et al. found an association in smokers who attended a vascular clinic. However, the risk odds ratio was much higher for those with peripheral arterial disease (4.8) compared to those who smoked (1.9) [40].

Outlook: Future Developments

The risk factors for relapse and reinfection are the same as the predisposing factors for onychomycosis [18]. However, the risk factors for dermatophytic infections are not the same as for mold onychomycosis. Moreover, no systemic or local predisposing factors for mold onychomycosis have been identified [48]. Important future directions will include recognizing any predisposing factors for mold onychomycosis, if they exist, as well as optimizing or personalizing treatment plans based on what underlying conditions and predisposing conditions patients have.

Summary for the Clinician
Predisposing factors for onychomycosis include genetic, medical, physical, and environmental factors. Certain comorbid medical conditions such as diabetes or an immunosuppressed state are especially associated with a higher prevalence of onychomycosis. Further, treatment for patients with certain diseases or physical characteristics, like diabetes and obesity, may be less effective. Identification and management of these underlying conditions is important.

References

1. Summerbell RC, Kane J, Krajden S. Onychomycosis, tinea pedis and tinea manuum caused by non-dermatophytic filamentous fungi. Mycoses. 1989;32(12):609–19.
2. Caputo R, De Boulle K, Del Rosso J, Nowicki R. Prevalence of superficial fungal infections among sports-active individuals: results from the Achilles survey, a review of the literature. J Eur Acad Dermatol Venereol (JEADV). 2001;15(4):312–6.
3. Elewski BE, Charif MA. Prevalence of onychomycosis in patients attending a dermatology clinic in northeastern Ohio for other conditions. Arch Dermatol. 1997;133(9):1172–3.
4. Heikkila H, Stubb S. The prevalence of onychomycosis in Finland. Br J Dermatol. 1995;133(5):699–703.
5. Sais G, Jucgla A, Peyri J. Prevalence of dermatophyte onychomycosis in Spain: a cross-sectional study. Br J Dermatol. 1995;132(5):758–61.
6. Ghannoum MA, Hajjeh RA, Scher R, et al. A large-scale North American study of fungal isolates from nails: the frequency of onychomycosis, fungal distribution, and antifungal susceptibility patterns. J Am Acad Dermatol. 2000;43(4):641–8.
7. Pierard G. Onychomycosis and other superficial fungal infections of the foot in the elderly: a pan-European survey. Dermatology. 2001;202(3):220–4.
8. Elewski BE, Tosti A. Risk factors and comorbidities for onychomycosis: implications for treatment with topical therapy. J Clin Aesthet Dermatol. 2015;8(11):38–42.
9. Belyayeva E, Gregoriou S, Chalikias J, et al. The impact of nail disorders on quality of life. Eur J Dermatol (EJD). 2013;23(3):366–71.
10. Schein JR, Gause D, Stier DM, Lubeck DP, Bates MM, Fisk R. Onychomycosis. Baseline results of an observational study. J Am Podiatr Med Assoc. 1997;87(11):512–9.
11. Milobratovic D, Jankovic S, Vukicevic J, Marinkovic J, Jankovic J, Railic Z. Quality of life in patients with toenail onychomycosis. Mycoses. 2013;56(5):543–51.
12. Papini M, Piraccini BM, Difonzo E, Brunoro A. Epidemiology of onychomycosis in Italy: prevalence data and risk factor identification. Mycoses. 2015;58(11):659–64.
13. Sigurgeirsson B, Steingrimsson O. Risk factors associated with onychomycosis. J Eur Acad Dermatol Venereol (JEADV). 2004;18(1):48–51.
14. Polat M, Ilhan MN. Dermatological complaints of the elderly attending a dermatology outpatient clinic in Turkey: a prospective study over a one-year period. Acta Dermatovenerol Croat (ADC). 2015;23(4):277–81.
15. Deo MS, Kerse N, Vandal AC, Jarrett P. Dermatological disease in the older age group: a cross-sectional study in aged care facilities. BMJ Open. 2015;5(12):e009941.

16. Gupta AK, Sibbald RG, Lynde CW, et al. Onychomycosis in children: prevalence and treatment strategies. J Am Acad Dermatol. 1997;36(3 Pt 1):395–402.
17. Gupta C, Das S, Ramachandran VG, et al. Possible role of trichophytin antigen in inducing impaired immunological clearance of fungus in onychomycosis. Mycopathologia. 2016; 181(3–4):247–51.
18. Tosti A, Hay R, Arenas-Guzman R. Patients at risk of onychomycosis–risk factor identification and active prevention. J Eur Acad Dermatol Venereol (JEADV). 2005;19(Suppl 1):13–6.
19. Zaias N, Tosti A, Rebell G, et al. Autosomal dominant pattern of distal subungual onychomycosis caused by Trichophyton rubrum. J Am Acad Dermatol. 1996;34(2 Pt 1):302–4.
20. English MP. Trichophyton rubrum infection in families. Br Med J. 1957;1(5021):744–6.
21. Many H, Derbes VJ, Friedman L. Trichophyton rubrum: exposure and infection within household groups. Arch Dermatol. 1960;82:226–9.
22. Zaitz C, Campbell I, Moraes JR, et al. HLA-associated susceptibility to chronic onychomycosis in Brazilian Ashkenazic Jews. Int J Dermatol. 1996;35(9):681–2.
23. Asz-Sigall D, Lopez-Garcia L, Vega-Memije ME, et al. HLA-DR6 association confers increased resistance to *T. rubrum* onychomycosis in Mexican Mestizos. Int J Dermatol. 2010;49(12):1406–9.
24. Svejgaard E, Jakobsen B, Svejgaard A. HLA studies in chronic dermatophytosis caused by Trichophyton rubrum. Acta Derm Venereol. 1983;63(3):254–5.
25. Zuccarello D, Salpietro DC, Gangemi S, et al. Familial chronic nail candidiasis with ICAM-1 deficiency: a new form of chronic mucocutaneous candidiasis. J Med Genet. 2002;39(9): 671–5.
26. Ferwerda B, Ferwerda G, Plantinga TS, et al. Human dectin-1 deficiency and mucocutaneous fungal infections. N Engl J Med. 2009;361(18):1760–7.
27. Gupta AK, Konnikov N, MacDonald P, et al. Prevalence and epidemiology of toenail onychomycosis in diabetic subjects: a multicentre survey. Br J Dermatol. 1998;139(4):665–71.
28. Dogra S, Kumar B, Bhansali A, Chakrabarty A. Epidemiology of onychomycosis in patients with diabetes mellitus in India. Int J Dermatol. 2002;41(10):647–51.
29. Elbendary A, El Tawdy A, Zaki N, Alfishawy M, Rateb A. Subclinical onychomycosis in patients with type II diabetes. Dermatol Reports. 2015;7(3):6099.
30. Papini M, Cicoletti M, Fabrizi V, Landucci P. Skin and nail mycoses in patients with diabetic foot. G Ital Dermatol Venereol (Organo ufficiale, Societa italiana di dermatologia e sifilografia). 2013;148(6):603–8.
31. Wijesuriya TM, Kottahachchi J, Gunasekara TD, et al. Aspergillus species: an emerging pathogen in onychomycosis among diabetics. Indian J Endocrinol Metab. 2015;19(6):811–6.
32. Vlahovic TC, Joseph WS. Efinaconazole topical, 10 % for the treatment of toenail onychomycosis in patients with diabetes. J Drugs Dermatol (JDD). 2014;13(10):1186–90.
33. Gupta AK, Taborda P, Taborda V, et al. Epidemiology and prevalence of onychomycosis in HIV-positive individuals. Int J Dermatol. 2000;39(10):746–53.
34. Cribier B, Mena ML, Rey D, et al. Nail changes in patients infected with human immunodeficiency virus. A prospective controlled study. Arch Dermatol. 1998;134(10):1216–20.
35. Gianni C, Cerri A, Capsoni F, Ongari AM, Rossini P, Crosti C. Recurrent proximal white subungual onychomycosis associated with a defect of the polymorphonuclear chemotaxis. Eur J Dermatol (EJD). 1999;9(5):390–2.
36. Walling HW. Subclinical onychomycosis is associated with tinea pedis. Br J Dermatol. 2009;161(4):746–9.
37. Staberg B, Gammeltoft M, Onsberg P. Onychomycosis in patients with psoriasis. Acta Derm Venereol. 1983;63(5):436–8.
38. Gupta AK, Lynde CW, Jain HC, et al. A higher prevalence of onychomycosis in psoriatics compared with non-psoriatics: a multicentre study. Br J Dermatol. 1997;136(5):786–9.
39. Larsen GK, Haedersdal M, Svejgaard EL. The prevalence of onychomycosis in patients with psoriasis and other skin diseases. Acta Derm Venereol. 2003;83(3):206–9.

40. Gupta AK, Gupta MA, Summerbell RC, et al. The epidemiology of onychomycosis: possible role of smoking and peripheral arterial disease. J Eur Acad Dermatol Venereol (JEADV). 2000;14(6):466–9.
41. Ozkan F, Ozturk P, Ozyurt K, et al. Frequency of peripheral arterial disease and venous insufficiency in toenail onychomycosis. J Dermatol. 2013;40(2):107–10.
42. Saez de Ocariz MM, Arenas R, Ranero-Juarez GA, Farrera-Esponda F, Monroy-Ramos E. Frequency of toenail onychomycosis in patients with cutaneous manifestations of chronic venous insufficiency. Int J Dermatol. 2001;40(1):18–25.
43. Fukunaga A, Washio K, Ogura K, et al. Onychomycosis as a warning sign for peripheral arterial disease. Acta Derm Venereol. 2013;93(6):747–8.
44. Eisele SA. Conditions of the toenails. Orthop Clin North Am. 1994;25(1):183–8.
45. Gudnadottir G, Hilmarsdottir I, Sigurgeirsson B. Onychomycosis in Icelandic swimmers. Acta Derm Venereol. 1999;79(5):376–7.
46. Nurhan Doner SY. Tugba Rezan Emekci Evaluation of Obesity-Associated Dermatoses in Obese and Overweight Individuals. Turkderm. 2011;45(3):146–51.
47. Bandh SA, Kamili AN, Ganai BA, Lone BA. Opportunistic fungi in lake water and fungal infections in associated human population in Dal Lake, Kashmir. Microb Pathog. 2016;93:105–10.
48. Tosti A, Piraccini BM, Lorenzi S. Onychomycosis caused by nondermatophytic molds: clinical features and response to treatment of 59 cases. J Am Acad Dermatol. 2000;42(2 Pt 1): 217–24.

Chapter 3
Distal Subungual Onychomycosis

Jeremy Brandon Freedman and Antonella Tosti

Key Features

- More than 85 % of all fungal nail infections (onychomycosis) present as distal lateral subungual onychomycosis (DLSO).
- Major predisposing factors are age, diabetes, and peripheral vascular disease.
- The general clinical presentation of DLSO is discoloration of the nail, subungual hyperkeratosis, and onycholysis.
- DLSO is easy to confuse with other nail dystrophies that mimic its appearance (i.e., trauma, psoriasis, lichen planus, etc.). Therefore, KOH, fungal culture, or PAS stain is necessary to confirm the diagnosis.
- Recurrence and reinfection are common.

Introduction

Distal lateral subungual onychomycosis (DLSO) is the single most common form of fungal nail infection and accounts for approximately 41 % of *all* nail abnormalities [1]. It is classically characterized by fungal invasion of the nail bed from under the free edge of the nail (the hyponychium), often as an extension of tinea pedis (Fig. 3.1). This causes subungual hyperkeratosis, thickening and discoloration of the nail plate, and eventual onycholysis (detachment of the nail from the nail bed).

Although not life threatening, these ugly, unsightly nails are evidence of a deceptively complex condition that can cause considerable pain and make it difficult to

J.B. Freedman, BA • A. Tosti (✉)
Department of Dermatology and Cutaneous Surgery,
University of Miami Miller School of Medicine, Miami, FL 33136, USA
e-mail: JBFreedman@miami.edu; atosti@med.miami.edu

A. Tosti et al. (eds.), *Onychomycosis*, DOI 10.1007/978-3-319-44853-4_3

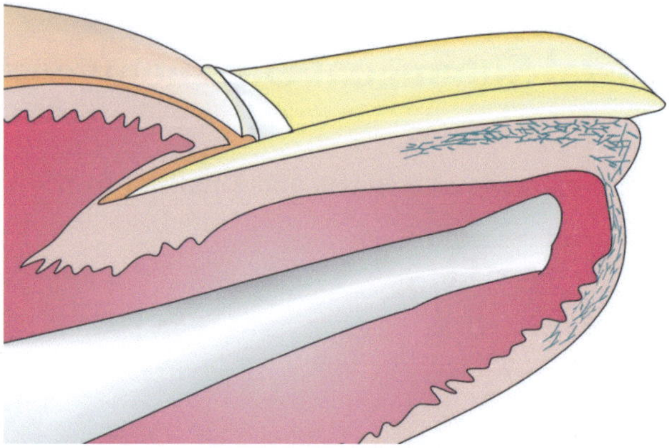

Fig. 3.1 This schematic illustrates the progression of fungal infection in DLSO, specifically how the fungus gains access to the nail bed via the hyponychium

perform simple daily activities like walking and wearing shoes. Additionally, if allowed to progress, DLSO can cause significant complications, including bacterial superinfection and cellulitis.

Aside from the physical symptoms, it's also important to keep in mind the powerful psychosocial impact DLSO can have on quality of life. Many patients report feelings of severe embarrassment over the appearance of their fungal nails, problems with self-esteem, and social withdrawal [4, 5]. Recent surveys confirm that people who suffer from onychomycosis are more likely to be excluded from social activities, and are perceived by others as less likely to be able to form good relationships as well as less likely to succeed at work [6].

Sadly, despite the potential complications and obviously diseased appearance of infected nails, DLSO is often dismissed as "merely" a cosmetic problem and is commonly ignored or incompletely treated. This may have something to do with the fact that fungal infections of the nail are notoriously difficult to cure, partially due to factors inherent to the nail itself: the sluggish growth of the nail means diseased portions are slow to be replaced, and the hard, protective nail plate inhibits topical drugs from reaching the fungal pathogens on the nail bed beneath it. Also, patients are regularly plagued with recurrences and reinfections [2, 7], and, faced with a choice between oral systemic medications requiring laboratory monitoring for toxicity, or lengthy topical therapies that often require nail debridement and multiple return visits, many patients are – unsurprisingly – noncompliant. This further complicates the course of the disease.

Although DLSO can occur in either the fingernails, toenails, or both, toenails are overwhelmingly more often affected, with a toenail to fingernail ratio of 19:1 [1]. The vast majority of toenail fungal infections (greater than 90 % of cases) are caused by dermatophytes (parasitic fungal organisms that feed on keratin), but they can less frequently be caused by non-dermatophytic molds and yeasts. The causal organisms of fingernail onychomycosis are almost exclusively dermatophytes.

Epidemiology

Unfortunately, it's difficult to quantify the exact prevalence of DLSO, as estimates vary widely from study to study (ranging from 2 to 13 %) [1, 8–15]. This is partly because DLSO (and onychomycosis in general) is highly dependent on geographic location, and partly due to differences in study methodology, like the population source (e.g., were they patients who presented with nail complaints, or simply those in for regular checkups?). As a matter of fact, some have even suggested that – while it is undeniably common – the general prevalence of fungal nail infections has been slightly overestimated by hospital-based studies [10].

That being said, there has *clearly* been a steady upward trend in the past few decades. In 1979, a population study in North America reported the prevalence of onychomycosis to be just over 2 % [16]. Less than 20 years later, that number had jumped to more than 8.5 % [8]. More recently, a large multicenter study reported it to be 13.8 % [9]. Considering that DLSO accounts for greater than 85 % of all onychomycosis cases, this directly translates into a rising incidence of DLSO. This burgeoning growth can be tied to changes in the culture of modern society, first among them an increase in our use of occlusive footwear which provides a warm, moist, confined environment that is highly conducive to fungal growth. Onychomycosis prevalence (and, by extension, DLSO) has actually been shown to decrease in populations wearing nonocclusive footwear, like sandals [17]. Another factor in the spread of fungal infections like DLSO is the increasing popularity of public pools, fitness center locker rooms, etc., where wet floors provide favorable breeding grounds for fungi and people are often barefoot [18].

Multiple studies have noted that family members of patients infected with DLSO have a higher risk of contracting the disease [19]. Initially, it was believed that this higher risk was *solely* due to intrafamilial transmission, i.e., increased exposure to a reservoir of infection. However, more recent studies have indicated that DLSO has a genetic component: susceptibility to infection by *Trichophyton rubrum* appears to be inherited in an autosomal dominant pattern [20, 21]. Subsequent studies identified specific genotypes affecting the immune system that prevent "the production of a full adaptive immune response," leaving these individuals susceptible to fungal overgrowth and chronic infections [22].

Additionally, several studies have observed that men are almost three times more likely to develop onychomycosis than women [23]. Although the reasons for this gender difference aren't fully understood, it likely involves social and/or genetic factors.

Aside from culture, environment, and genetics, the greatest predisposing risk factor for DLSO appears to be advanced age, as several studies have shown an increased prevalence of onychomycosis with increasing age [1, 3]. The rate of fungal nail infections in the general population is approximately 10 %, but in adults over age 70, that number can climb as high as 50 % [2, 3]. This is most likely explained by the fact that the nail grows slower with aging and infection can progress easily. Common comorbidities seen in the elderly are also risk factors for

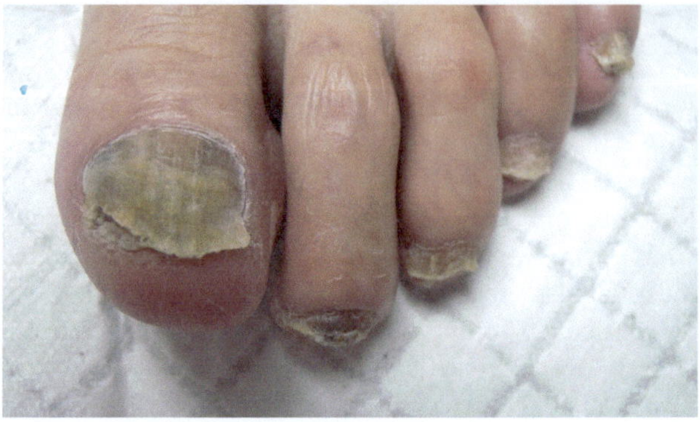

Fig. 3.2 DLSO in a diabetic patient. All nails are affected. Note the tinea pedis scaling and the hematoma of the great toe (due to poor fitting shoes, which is common due to neuropathy)

DLSO, including poor peripheral circulation, diabetes, decreased immune function, repeated nail trauma, longer exposure to pathogenic fungi, and even the simple inability to maintain good foot care.

It's therefore unsurprising that children are rarely affected by DLSO. A prospective, multicenter survey found the prevalence of fungal nail infections in North American children 18 years old or younger to be less than .5 % [24]. Aside from the fact that there is a relative absence of the previously listed common DLSO risk factors in young people, reasons for the incredibly low infection rate compared to adults can also be explained by their lower prevalence of tinea pedis, faster nail growth, and generally smaller nails, which provide less surface area for fungal invasion.

As mentioned, diabetes is a notable underlying comorbidity in patients with DLSO. Approximately one-third of diabetics have a fungal nail infection, and they are 2.77 times more likely to develop onychomycosis than their nondiabetic counterparts (Fig. 3.2) [23]. Also, their impaired wound healing and sensory neuropathy put them at higher risk for more serious, limb-threatening complications. The jagged edges of their thickened, brittle nails can injure the surrounding soft tissue and create an unnoticed entry point for bacteria, fungi, or other pathogens, resulting in significant infections that may eventually lead to the need for amputation [25]. Retrospective studies have determined that diabetics with fungal infections like DLSO are approximately 3–5 times more likely to develop foot ulcers and/or gangrene than diabetics without onychomycosis [26].

It's particularly important to keep in mind the relationship between DLSO and tinea pedis [7]. The same dermatophyte organism (*Trichophyton rubrum*) is the major cause of both fungal infections [10, 27], and therefore each condition can serve as a reservoir of infection for the other. That's why DLSO is almost always preceded (or accompanied) by an infection of tinea pedis (Fig. 3.3). This relationship partially explains the greatly increased frequency of toenail compared to fingernail DLSO: the greater incidence of tinea pedis over tinea manuum provides more opportunities for the toenails to be infected.

Of course, if patients scratch or pick at their fungally infected feet, toes, or toenails, it's possible for them to transfer the fungus onto their hands, which can cause

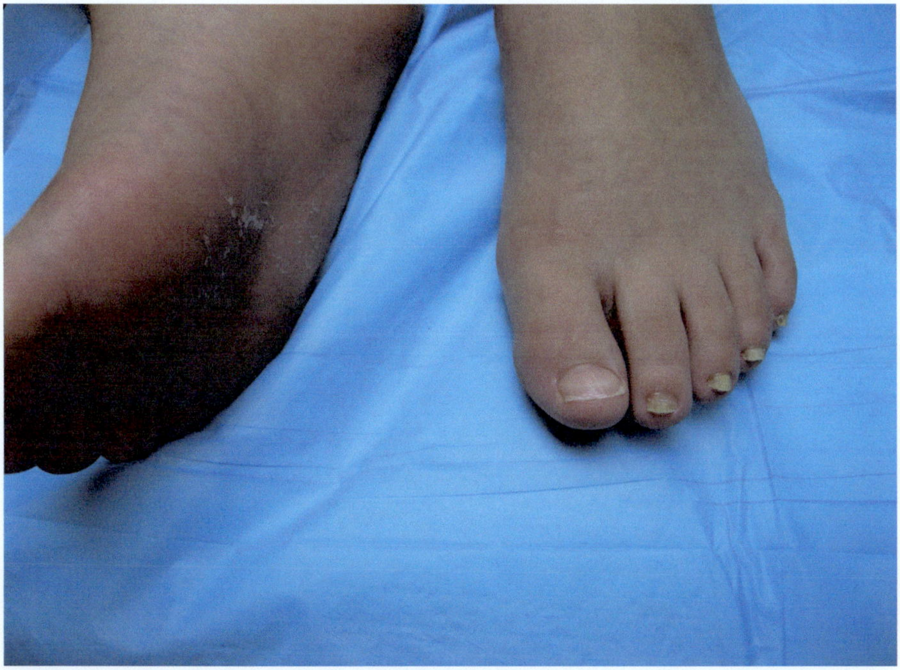

Fig. 3.3 DLSO and concomitant tinea pedis on the plantar surface of the opposite foot due to *T. rubrum*

Fig. 3.4 An example of fingernail DLSO

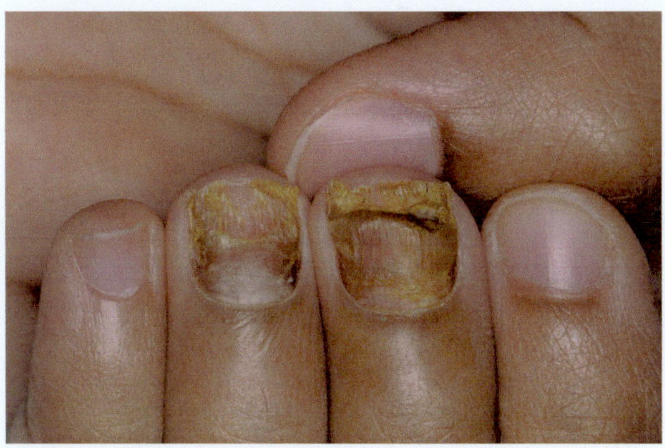

them to develop tinea manuum and/or fingernail DLSO (Fig. 3.4). This often causes the patient to develop a relatively common pattern of infection known as "two feet-one hand syndrome (Fig. 3.5)" [28, 29].

Overall, the incidence of DLSO is projected to continue increasing, largely due to a surge in critical risk factors like the age of the population, along with an increased prevalence of diabetes and peripheral vascular disease.

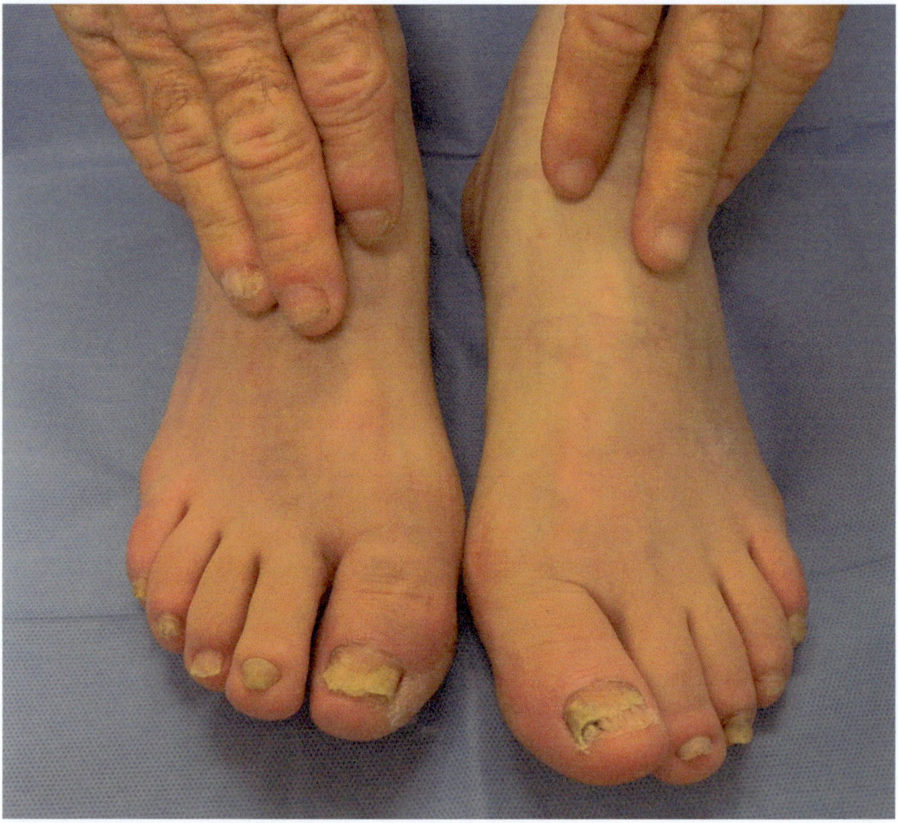

Fig. 3.5 DLSO is present on the nails of both feet and the right hand, while the left hand is unaffected (two feet-one hand syndrome)

Clinical Features

The characteristic features of DLSO are discoloration of the nail, subungual hyperkeratosis, and onycholysis (Fig. 3.6).

True to its name, DLSO's fungal organism invades the nail bed at the distal portion of the nail. The fungus usually first infects the palm or sole, causing tinea pedis or tinea manuum, and then spreads from the skin to the nail bed via the hyponychium or the lateral nail fold.

In the early stages of infection, the fungus is limited to the nail bed, and the nail plate may appear normal. During this time, the stratum corneum of the nail bed often begins to thicken (subungual hyperkeratosis) due to mild inflammation from the fungal infection. The resulting keratotic debris pushes the nail plate up, eventually causing onycholysis.

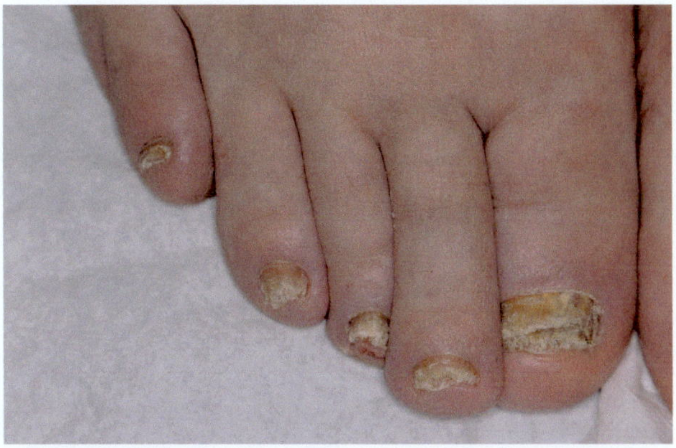

Fig. 3.6 DSLO. Note the yellow discoloration, severe subungual hyperkeratosis, and onycholysis

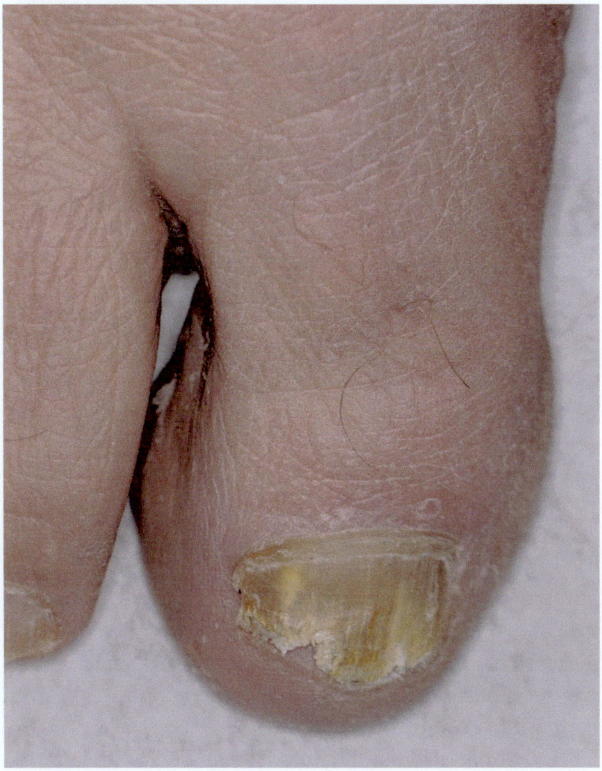

Fig. 3.7 The proximal progression of the fungus causes the yellow streaks leading toward the proximal nail fold. Also, note the tinea pedis scaling

From the initial site of infection, fungi migrate proximally (toward the cuticle) along the longitudinally oriented rete ridges of the nail bed. This explains the yellow, orange, or white longitudinal spikes and streaks which are a typical sign of progressing disease (Figs. 3.7 and 3.8).

The nail plate may also display diffuse discoloration and look yellow, orange, or white. Less commonly, when DLSO is caused by non-dermatophytic fungal molds that produce melanin, the nail presents with a brown/black pigmentation (ungual

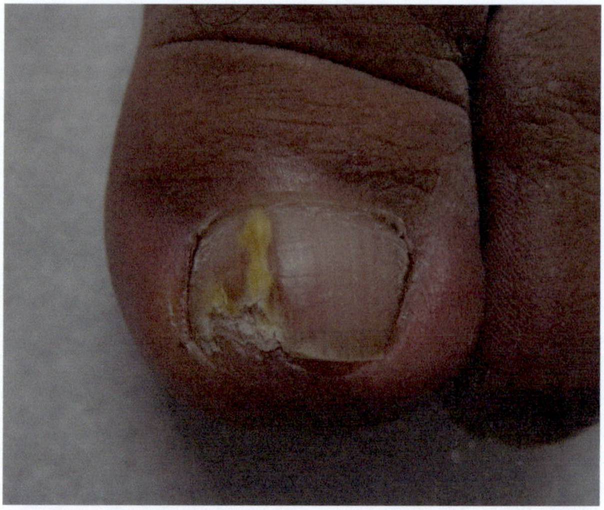

Fig. 3.8 Another example of a discolored longitudinal streak due to proximal fungal progression, this one extending all the way into the lunula. There is also subungual hyperkeratosis

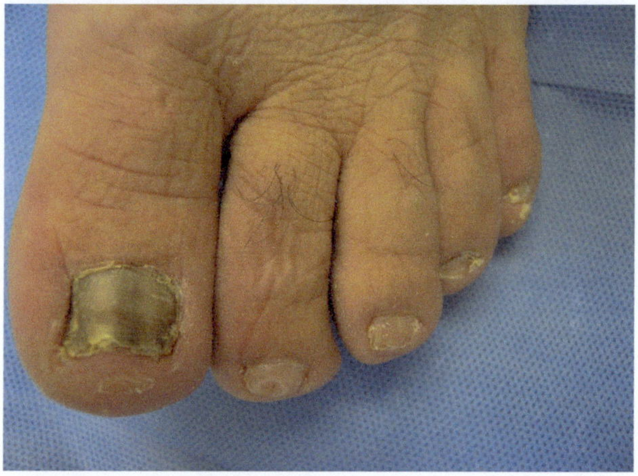

Fig. 3.9 Pigmented DLSO

melanonychia) similar in appearance to nail melanoma (Fig. 3.9). Thankfully, this is relatively rare, as many of the organisms which cause ungual melanonychia (e.g., *Neoscytalidium dimidiatum*) do not respond to antifungal therapies and are very difficult to cure [30].

Sometimes dermatophytomas (rounded or linear areas of particularly dense discoloration) are observed (Figs. 3.10 and 3.11a,b). This is generally a more advanced form of the disease and is considered a negative prognostic factor. A dermatophytoma indicates a fungal abscess (a mass of hyphae and spores) under the nail. The fungi in these masses create a biofilm and are particularly difficult to treat without debridement.

In time DLSO can progress to total dystrophic onychomycosis (TDO) characterized by a thickened and crumbled dystrophic nail. However, as patients often cut the detached nail plate, particularly in fingernails, clinical presentation can be less typical (Fig. 3.12).

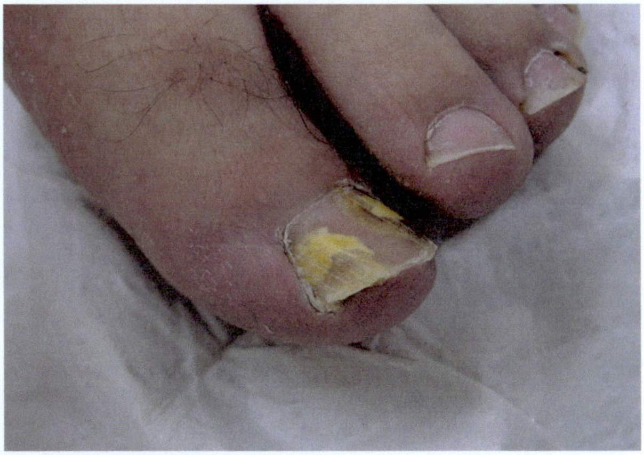

Fig. 3.10 Note the prominent dermatophytomas on the great toe

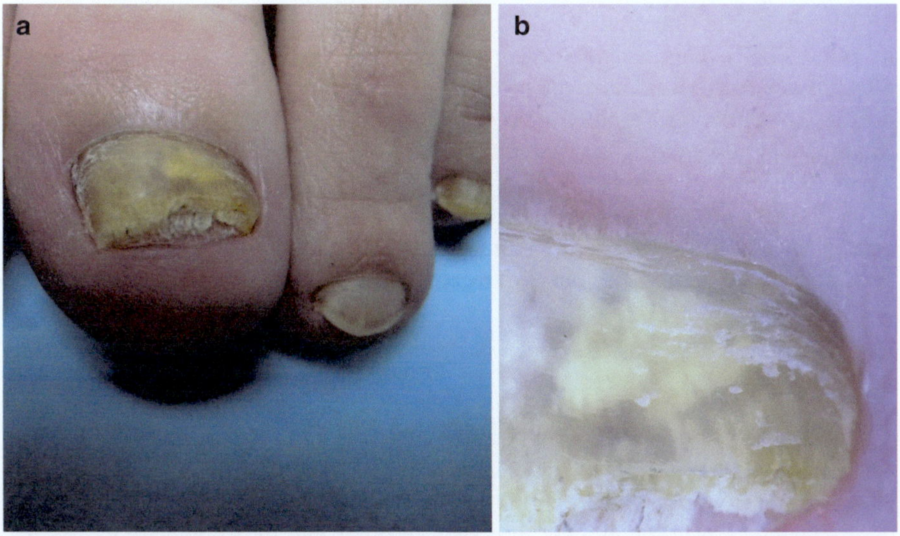

Fig. 3.11 (**a**, **b**) Nail discoloration, subungual hyperkeratosis, onycholysis, and a dermatophytoma (**a**). A dermatoscopic image of a patch that doesn't reach the free margin of the nail (**b**)

Several specific clinical findings are considered factors that predict a poor response to treatment. These include dermatophytomas, cases where greater than 50 % of the nail is affected (especially if there is significant involvement of the lateral nail), cases with more than 2 mm of subungual hyperkeratosis, as well as those cases where the disease has progressed to TDO with matrix involvement. Other negative prognostic factors have to do with the fungal organism itself (e.g., a *Neoscytalidium* mold, as discussed above) or are patient specific – those with immunosuppression or diminished peripheral circulation have a higher likelihood of treatment failure.

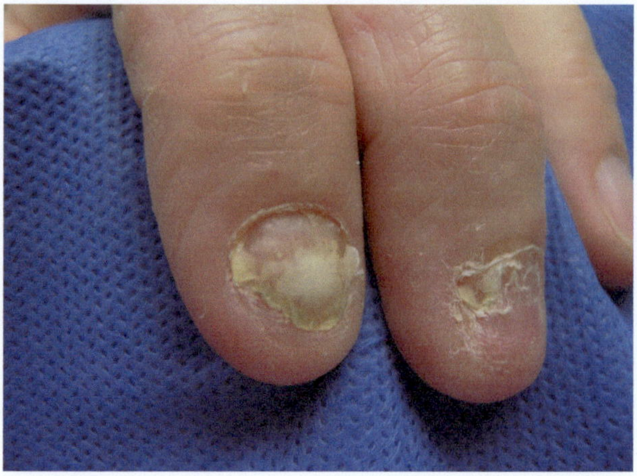

Fig. 3.12 Fingernail DLSO where the patient cut the affected nail

The severity of infection can also be determined using the onychomycosis severity index (OSI). This simple scoring system takes into account the percentage of affected onychomycotic nail, the proximity of infection to the nail matrix, and the presence of either dermatophytomas, longitudinal streaks, or greater than 2 mm of subungual hyperkeratosis, and calculates a score from 1 to 35. Mild disease is classified by a score of 5 or below, moderate disease by 6–15, and severe disease by 6–35 [31]. By providing an objective measurement of disease severity that can be quickly assessed as the clinical picture changes, patients can be followed more accurately throughout their course of treatment.

Diagnostic Clues

Making a conclusive clinical diagnosis of DLSO can be difficult, as many of its classic features (nail discoloration, subungual hyperkeratosis, onycholysis, and thick, damaged, brittle nails) are also seen in other nail dystrophies (e.g., trauma, psoriasis, lichen planus, onychogryphosis, etc.). However, the mechanisms of fungal progression provide plenty of clinical signs that can suggest a diagnosis of DLSO and indicate the need for further confirmatory laboratory testing.

As the fungus usually first infects the palm or sole and only then spreads to the nail bed, first inspect the skin on the soles, fingertips, and between the toes for signs of tinea pedis/tinea manuum scaling. While the absence of scaling doesn't necessarily rule out a diagnosis of DLSO, its presence can help in making a positive diagnosis.

Once the fungus invades the nail bed and the stratum corneum begins to thicken, subungual hyperkeratosis causes onycholysis. The keratotic debris lifting the nail creates a unique appearance under the free edge of the nail that De Crignis et al. call "ruin appearance" [32]. By inspecting the hyponychium with a dermatoscope, this

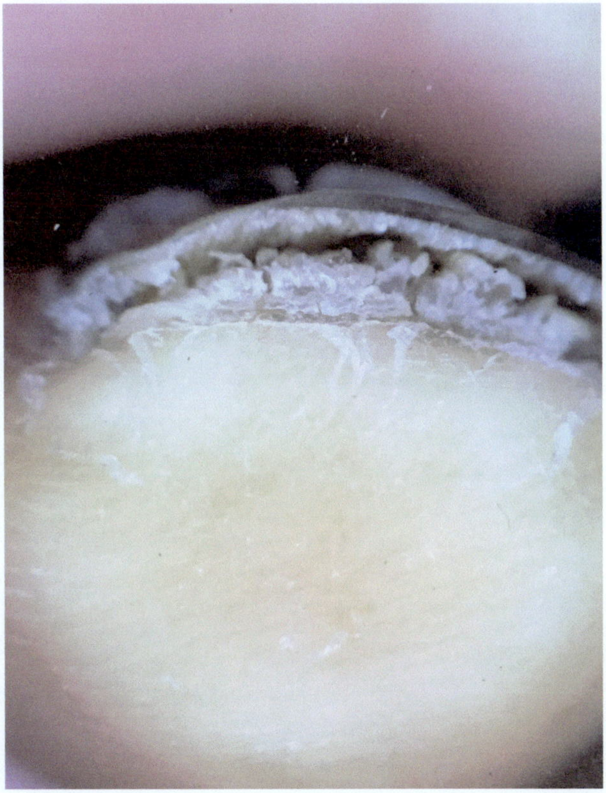

Fig. 3.13 A dermatoscopic image of the distal border of the nail showing "ruin appearance"

appearance can be clearly visualized (Fig. 3.13). Again, the absence of ruin appearance doesn't necessarily rule out a diagnosis of DLSO; however, its presence is *very* indicative of a positive diagnosis.

As the fungus advances longitudinally along the rete ridges of the nail bed, it causes a specific longitudinal pattern of discoloration which provides an easy, noninvasive method to differentiate between DLSO and conditions which merely mimic the appearance of DLSO, e.g., traumatic onycholysis, the second most common nail dystrophy. When examining the nail, use a dermatoscope to inspect the most proximal edge of the discolored/onycholytic area for an uneven border with sharp projections towards the proximal nail fold (Fig. 3.14). This visual cue (dubbed by Piraccini et al. as a "jagged edge with spikes") is distinct and exclusive to DLSO thanks to the behavior of the migrating fungus. Traumatic onycholysis presents with a smooth, linear edge without indentations [33, 34].

Another dermatoscopic finding caused by the proximally migrating fungus is an irregular matte pigmentation distributed in longitudinal striae on the detached nail plate. Since it forms a pattern similar to an aurora borealis, it was labeled by Piraccini et al. as an "Aurora Pattern." Its presence is also highly suggestive of DLSO [33].

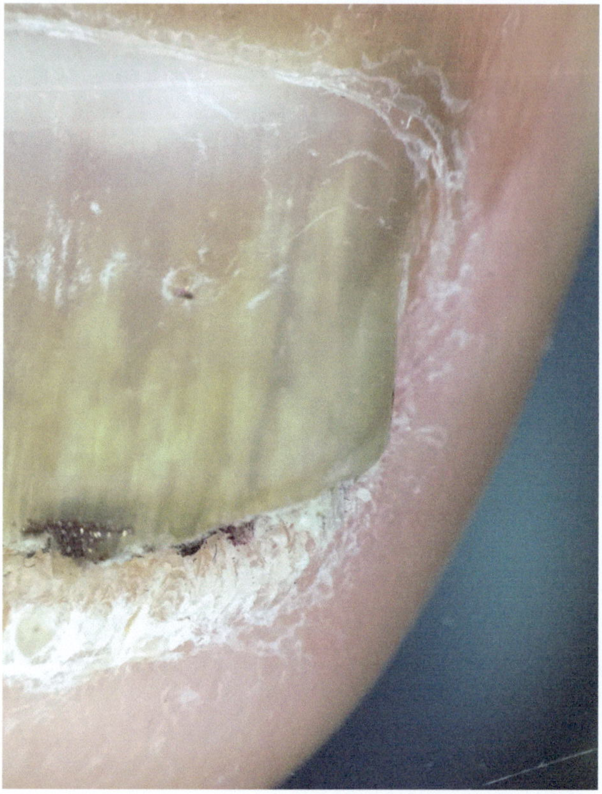

Fig. 3.14 A dermatoscopic image exhibiting "spikes" on the proximal margin, imbuing it with the "jagged edge" appearance

Summary for the Clinician

DLSO is incredibly common and can cause significant physical and psychosocial problems. Due to increasing incidence of important risk factors, we expect to see a concomitant increase in DLSO cases in the years to come.

Since only about half of all nail abnormalities can be attributed to fungal infections, it's important to be able to distinguish between true DLSO and other conditions that merely mimic its appearance before beginning treatment – which can be long, difficult, and expensive.

Unfortunately, the close similarities between many of the nail dystrophies tend to make obtaining a definitive clinical diagnosis very challenging. Therefore, while the clinical presentation combined with dermoscopy and a suggestive history can strongly point you in the direction of DLSO, the diagnosis needs to be confirmed by laboratory techniques [35].

Today, that means KOH, fungal culture, or a PAS stain. In the future, however, newer PCR techniques will probably be utilized more often, as they have advantages over all of those methods: PCR is faster (results are returned in days vs. weeks), unaffected by fungal viability, and is less susceptible to contamination.

Another reliable method is the dermatophyte test strip, shown to have an overall concordance rate of 95 % [36]. Keep in mind that these test strips will only identify dermatophyte infections, but those do account for the vast majority of onychomycosis cases.

Clinical Pearls

- If you see tinea pedis, look for onychomycosis.
- If someone comes in with fingernail disease, look at his or her toenails, and vice versa.
- Tell affected patients to put on their socks before their underwear to prevent transfer of fungus to the inguinal folds, causing tinea cruris.
- Although women and children have a lower incidence of infection, they are more likely to seek treatment. Ask them about other members of their family, as it's likely some will be infected.

References

1. Gupta AK, Jain HC, Lynde CW, et al. Prevalence and epidemiology of onychomycosis in patients visiting physicians' offices: a multicenter Canadian survey of 15,000 patients. J Am Acad Dermatol. 2000;43(2 Pt 1):244–8.
2. Rose AE. Therapeutic update: onychomycosis. J Drugs Dermatol. 2014;13(10):1173–5.
3. Thomas J, Jacobson GA, Narkowicz CK. Toenail onychomycosis: an important global disease burden. J Clin Pharm Ther. 2010;35(5):497–519.
4. Reich A, Szepietowski JC. Health-related quality of life in patients with nail disorders. Am J Clin Dermatol. 2011;12(5):313–20.
5. Chacon A, Franca K, Fernandez A, Nouri K. Psychosocial impact of onychomycosis: a review. Int J Dermatol. 2013;52(11):1300–7.
6. Chan HH, Wong ET, Yeung CK. Psychosocial perception of adults with onychomycosis: a blinded, controlled comparison of 1,017 adult Hong Kong residents with or without onychomycosis. Biopsychosoc Med. 2014;8:15.
7. Gupta AK, Elewski BE, Rosen T, et al. Onychomycosis: strategies to minimize recurrence. J Drugs Dermatol. 2016;15(3):279–82.
8. Elewski BE, Charif MA. Prevalence of onychomycosis in patients attending a dermatology clinic in northeastern Ohio for other conditions. Arch Dermatol. 1997;133(9):1172–3.
9. Ghannoum MA, Hajjeh RA, Scher R, et al. A large-scale North American study of fungal isolates from nails: the frequency of onychomycosis, fungal distribution, and antifungal susceptibility patterns. J Am Acad Dermatol. 2000;43(4):641–8.
10. Sigurgeirsson B, Baran R. The prevalence of onychomycosis in the global population: a literature study. J Eur Acad Dermatol Venereol. 2014;28(11):1480–91.
11. Heikkilä H, Stubb S. The prevalence of onychomycosis in Finland. Br J Dermatol. 1995;133(5):699–703.
12. Ioannidou DJ, Maraki S, Krasagakis SK, et al. The epidemiology of onychomycoses in Crete, Greece, between 1992 and 2001. J Eur Acad Dermatol Venereol. 2006;20(2):170–4.
13. Perea S, Ramos MJ, Garau M, et al. Prevalence and risk factors of tinea unguium and tinea pedis in the general population in Spain. J Clin Microbiol. 2000;38(9):3226–30.

14. Roberts DT. Prevalence of dermatophyte onychomycosis in the United Kingdom: results of an omnibus survey. Br J Dermatol. 1992;126(Suppl 39):23–7.
15. Svejgaard EL, Nilsson J. Onychomycosis in Denmark: prevalence of fungal nail infection in general practice. Mycoses. 2004;47(3–4):131–5.
16. Kraning KK, Odland GF. Prevalence, morbidity, and cost of dermatological diseases. J Invest Dermatol. 1979;73:395–401.
17. Nickerson WJ, Irving L, Mehmert HE. Sandals, and hygiene and infections of the feet. Arch Derm Syphilol. 1945;52:365–8.
18. Aly R. Ecology and epidemiology of dermatophyte infections. J Am Acad Dermatol. 1994;31(3 Pt 2):S21–5.
19. Many H, Derbes VJ, Friedman L. Trichophyton rubrum: exposure and infection within household groups. Arch Dermatol. 1960;82:226–9.
20. Zaias N, Tosti A, Rebell G, et al. Autosomal dominant pattern of distal subungual onychomycosis caused by Trichophyton rubrum. J Am Acad Dermatol. 1996;34(2 Pt 1):302–4.
21. Zaias N, Rebell G. Chronic dermatophytosis syndrome due to Trichophyton rubrum. Int J Dermatol. 1996;35(9):614–7.
22. Gupta AK, Simpson FC, Brintnell WC. Do genetic mutations and genotypes contribute to onychomycosis? Dermatology. 2014;228(3):207–10.
23. Gupta AK, Konnikov N, MacDonald P, et al. Prevalence and epidemiology of toenail onychomycosis in diabetic subjects: a multicentre survey. Br J Dermatol. 1998;139(4):665–71.
24. Gupta AK, Sibbald RG, Lynde CW, et al. Onychomycosis in children: prevalence and treatment strategies. J Am Acad Dermatol. 1997;36(3 Pt 1):395–402.
25. Brem H, Sheehan P, Boulton AJ. Protocol for treatment of diabetic foot ulcers. Am J Surg. 2004;187(5A):1S–10S.
26. Doyle JJ, Boyko WL, Ryu S, Gause D. Onychomycosis among diabetic patients: prevalence and impact of nonfungal foot infections [poster]. Presented at: The American Diabetes Association 60th Scientific Sessions; 2000; San Antonio, Tex. Reference ID: 104.
27. Foster KW, Ghannoum MA, Elewski BE. Epidemiologic surveillance of cutaneous fungal infection in the United States from 1999 to 2002. J Am Acad Dermatol. 2004;50(5):748–52.
28. Daniel 3rd CR, Gupta AK, Daniel MP, Daniel CM. Two feet-one hand syndrome: a retrospective multicenter survey. Int J Dermatol. 1997;36(9):658–60.
29. Zhan P, Ge YP, Lu XL, et al. A case-control analysis and laboratory study of the two feet-one hand syndrome in two dermatology hospitals in China. Clin Exp Dermatol. 2010;35(5):468–72.
30. Finch J, Arenas R, Baran R. Fungal melanonychia. J Am Acad Dermatol. 2012;66(5): 830–41.
31. Carney C, Tosti A, Daniel R, Scher R, Rich P, DeCoster J, Elewski B. A new classification system for grading the severity of onychomycosis: onychomycosis severity index. Arch Dermatol. 2011;147(11):1277–82.
32. De Crignis G, Valgas N, Rezende P, Leverone A, Nakamura R. Dermatoscopy of onychomycosis. Int J Dermatol. 2014;53(2):e97–9.
33. Piraccini BM, Balestri R, Starace M, Rech G. Nail digital dermoscopy (onychoscopy) in the diagnosis of onychomycosis. J Eur Acad Dermatol Venereol. 2013;27(4):509–13.
34. Jesús-Silva MA, Fernández-Martínez R, Roldán-Marín R, Arenas R. Dermoscopic patterns in patients with a clinical diagnosis of onychomycosis-results of a prospective study including data of potassium hydroxide (KOH) and culture examination. Dermatol Pract Concept. 2015;5(2):39–44.
35. Allevato MA. Diseases mimicking onychomycosis. Clin Dermatol. 2010;28(2):164–77.
36. Tsunemi Y, Hiruma M. Clinical study of Dermatophyte Test Strip, an immunochromatographic method, to detect tinea unguium dermatophytes. J Dermatol. 2016; doi:10.1111/1346-8138.13348.

Chapter 4
White Superficial Onychomycosis

Stephanie Mlacker and Antonella Tosti

> **Key Features**
> - In SWO the route of infection occurs via the dorsal aspect of the nail plate.
> - There are two variants of SWO: a superficial and a deep variant. SWO can rarely be pigmented. Rarely, SWO originates from beneath the proximal nail fold.
> - Deeper nail penetration has been linked to mold infection.
> - SWO is commonly associated with DLSO.
> - SWO can be treated with topical antifungals in most cases.

Introduction

Superficial white onychomycosis (SWO) refers to a form of onychomycosis that involves invasion of the nail plate through the dorsal surface (Fig. 4.1), presenting as opaque, friable, whitish superficial spots (Fig. 4.2) [1, 2]. However, this name is somewhat of a misnomer, as recent evidence supports a new classification of variants that includes a deep form of nail penetration. Organisms responsible for causing SWO include *Trichophyton mentagrophytes* var. *interdigitale*, which involves

S. Mlacker, BS (✉) • A. Tosti, MD
Department of Dermatology and Cutaneous Surgery, University of Miami Miller School of Medicine, 1475 NW 12th Ave., Suite 2175, Miami, FL 33136, USA
e-mail: mlackerstephanie@gmail.com; atosti@med.miami.edu

A. Tosti et al. (eds.), *Onychomycosis*, DOI 10.1007/978-3-319-44853-4_4

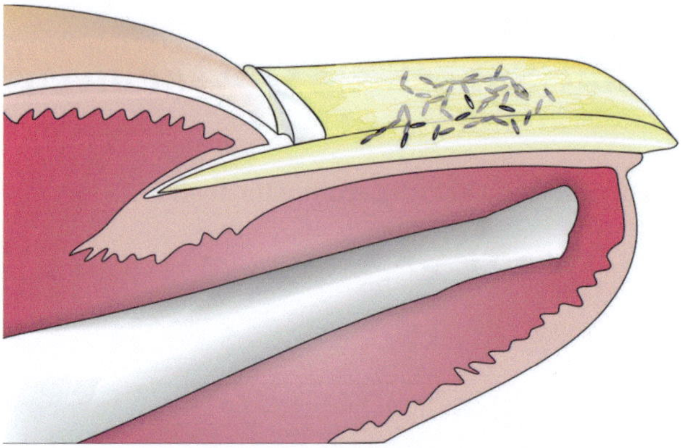

Fig. 4.1 SWO schematic drawing showing fungal invasion of the dorsal nail plate

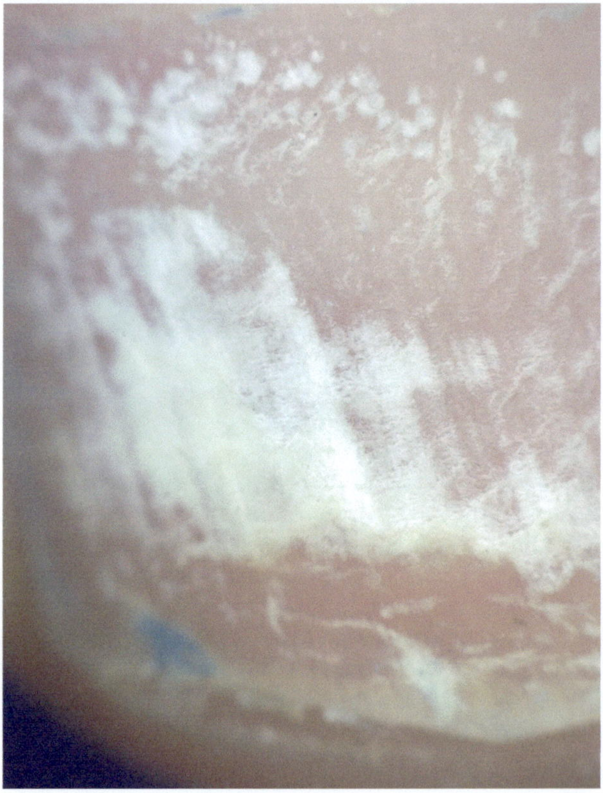

Fig. 4.2 SWO dermoscopy shows that the superficial nail plate is affected

90 % of cases, *Trichophyton rubrum*, or non-dermatophytes (molds), such as *Acremonium*, *Fusarium*, or *Aspergillus* species [1, 3, 4]. Infections from *Trichophyton rubrum* var. nigra or *Neoscytalidium dimidiatum* may cause "superficial black onychomycosis," when dark pigmentation is observed [5–7]. Of note, mixed

dermatophyte/non-dermatophyte infections may occur as well [8]. SWO usually affects the first, second, or third toenails. Fingernail involvement has rarely been reported in newborns or in HIV patients [7]. Toenails grow 50–66 % more slowly than fingernails, which can facilitate fungal infection [9]. Associated conditions include interdigital tinea pedis and, less frequently, plantar tinea pedis, both of which result from infection with *Trichophyton interdigitale* [7].

Epidemiology

Onychomycosis generally affects men more commonly than it affects women. Associated factors include diminished peripheral circulation, diabetes, trauma to the nail, and inadequate nail hygiene [10]. SWO is a rare type of onychomycosis that constitutes 1.5–7 % of all reported cases of fungal nail infections [11]. While SWO affects about 1–2 % of the general population, the incidence increases with age. Rate of prevalence is higher in the immunosuppressed, with 9.5 % of HIV-infected patients reportedly affected by SWO [7]. However, epidemiological characteristics may also vary according to the variant of SWO involved.

Clinical Features

There are two main subtypes of SWO: classical SWO and deep SWO (Figs. 4.3 and 4.4). In classical SWO, the superficial nail plate presents small white opaque friable patches with distinct borders. Scraping of the patches allows removal of the whitish surface material, exposing a transparent compact median nail plate. Sometimes, the patches may coalesce with time to involve the entire nail that becomes diffusely milky, white, and opaque [1, 3, 7]. One variant of classical SWO involves a route of infection that arises from below the proximal nail fold. This form of SWO, which may be difficult to distinguish from proximal subungual onychomycosis (PSO), most commonly affects children, who have thin nails, or immunosuppressed patients [1, 3]. In some cases, this variant presents with striate superficial bands, with affected white bands alternating with unaffected nail (Fig. 4.5). Deep invasion of the nail plate usually results from infection with non-dermatophytic molds, such as *Fusarium* and *Aspergillus* species, due to their eroding bodies which enable penetration of the nail plate barrier (Fig. 4.6) [4]. This deep variant is characterized by diffuse white and yellow-brown patches (Figs. 4.7 and 4.8). Nail plate discoloration may extend to the proximal nail fold, and the pigmentation can be visible through the cuticle [7]. Combination of SWO with another type of onychomycosis, such as distal and lateral subungual onychomycosis (DLSO) or proximal subungual onychomycosis (PSO), is not uncommon (Figs. 4.9 and 4.10) [1, 2].

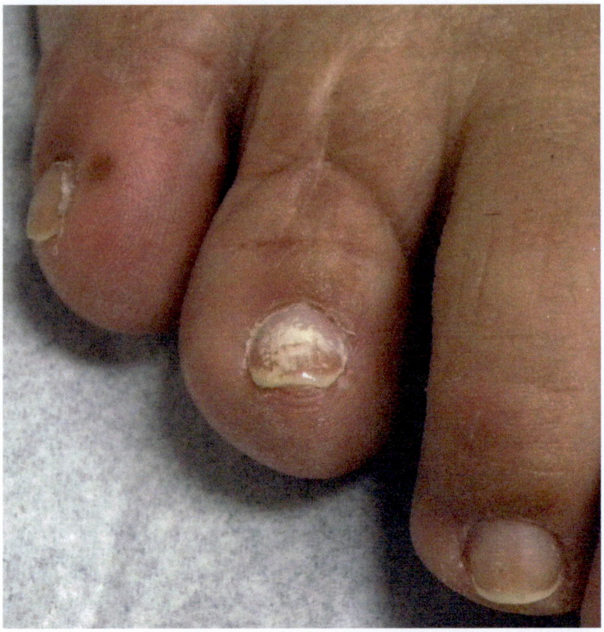

Fig. 4.3 SWO classical type

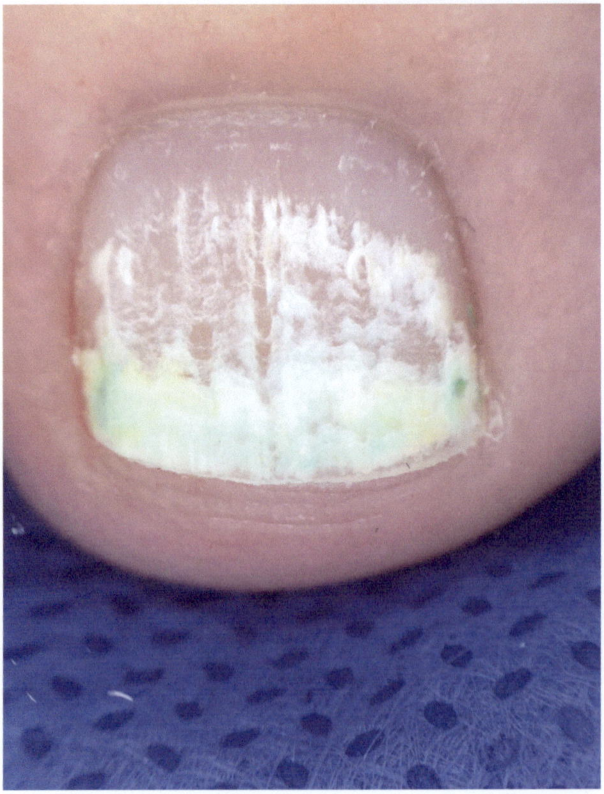

Fig. 4.4 Deep SWO

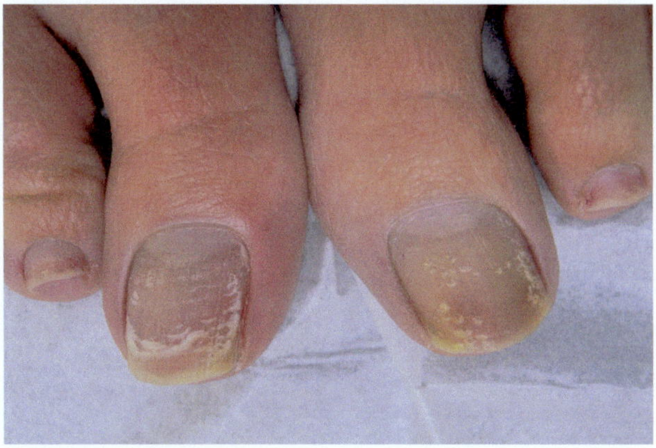

Fig. 4.5 SWO with striated pattern

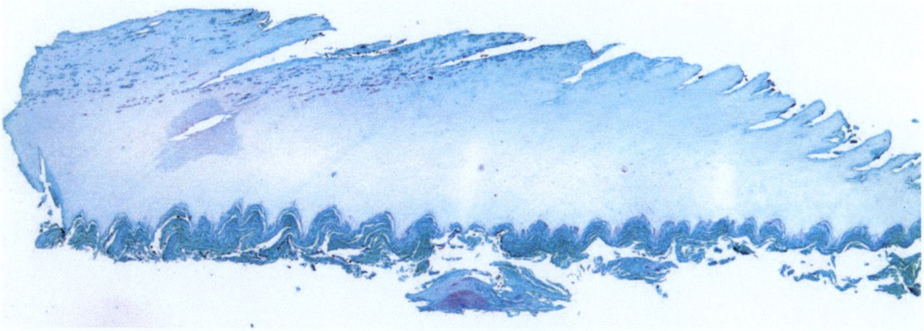

Fig. 4.6 Deep SWO: pathology shows fungal elements in the superficial and mid-nail plate

Diagnostic Clues

It is important to conduct mycological studies, in order to appropriately diagnose and treat onychomycosis [10]. Diagnosing SWO may be performed using direct microscopy with 40 % potassium hydroxide (KOH) mounts, fungal cultures, and nail clippings with periodic acid-Schiff (PAS) staining for histologic analysis (Fig. 4.11) [7, 12]. In some cases of SWO, taking a clipping might be difficult, as the infection is often located in the central part of the nail plate without involvement of the distal nail. Scraping of the superficial nail plate is the best way to obtain samples for KOH and culture. Of note, potassium hydroxide microscopy and culture carry a relatively low negative predictive value (<60 %) and, therefore, warrant repeat testing in patients with possible SWO that initially test negative [12].

When attempting to clinically distinguish the type of SWO involved, one can suspect a deeper invasion of the nail plate when scraping the dorsal surface fails to completely remove the white discoloration [3].

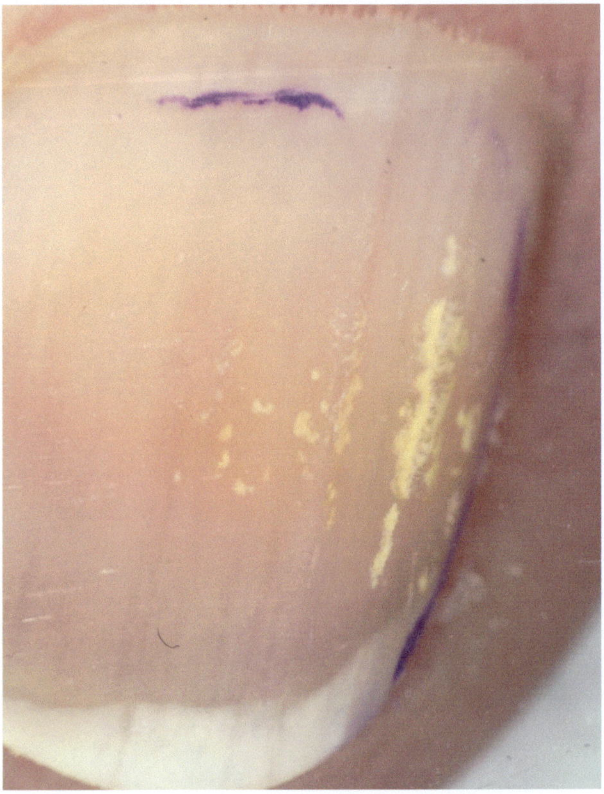

Fig. 4.7 SWO yellowish desquamating patch

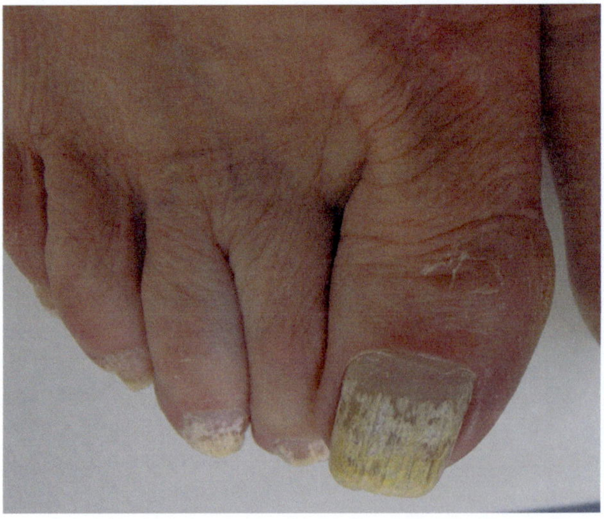

Fig. 4.8 SWO: note the yellow-white discoloration and crumbling of the nail surface

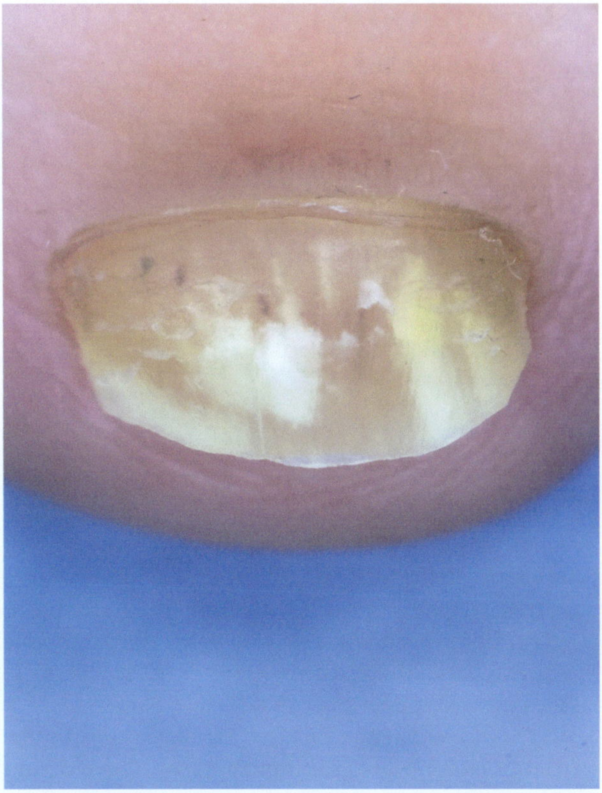

Fig. 4.9 SWO and DLSO affecting the same nail

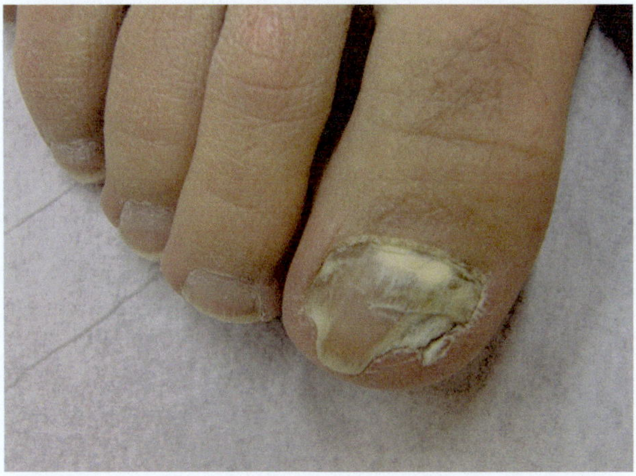

Fig. 4.10 SWO emerging from proximal nail fold and DLSO

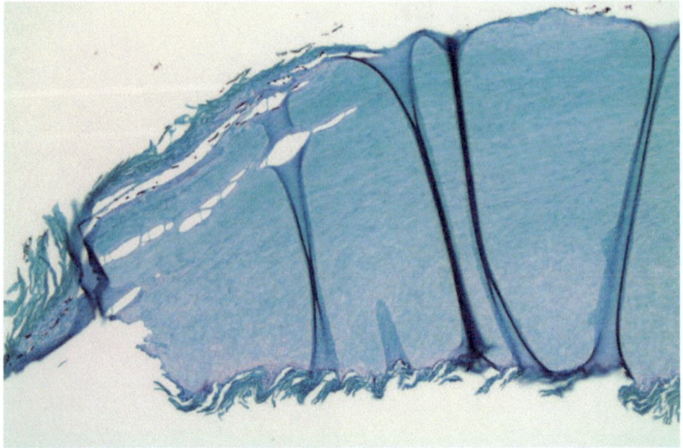

Fig. 4.11 SWO pathology shows fungal elements in the superficial nail plate

Summary for the Clinician

Clinicians must take into account features of both the host and causative organism in the treatment of patients with SWO. Dermatophytes contain keratolytic enzymes that allow them to break down the hard keratins of the nail plate. In vitro studies have shown the high osmotolerance characteristic of *T. interdigitale*, which contributes to its ability to invade the dry nail plate. However, it is important to note that SWO in HIV patients is commonly due to *T. rubrum* and may involve the fingernails. In the rare circumstances when *T. rubrum* is observed in immunocompetent individuals, it is usually the result of nail plate occlusion from an overriding toe. Other host factors involved in promoting SWO infections include diminished immune function, genetics, and nail plate thickness. For example, fungal invasion is more likely to involve the entire thickness of the nail plate in children who have thinner nails than adults. However, host factors are not likely implicated in SWO due to *Aspergillus* or *Fusarium*, as both species carry intrinsic properties that allow them to penetrate the nail's dorsal surface with greater depth and the affected hosts are typically healthy [7].

First-line treatment depends on the variant of SWO and generally entails mechanical removal, followed by administration of topical antifungals, with systemic antifungal agents, such as terbinafine or itraconazole, reserved for patients resistant to topical agents for more than 6 months [7, 11]. However, topical therapy is usually ineffective when the infection originates from beneath the proximal nail fold. It should be reserved for the classical variant of SWO, in which infection remains at a superficial level [5]. Systemic antifungal agents may be used either alone or in combination with topical antifungal, when the infection originates from below the proximal nail fold, when there is deep invasion or when there is a combination of variants present [1, 5].

Those infections emerging from below the proximal nail fold can share a similar fungal etiology as PSO, and therefore warrant close inspection. When clinicians isolate *T. rubrum* or *Fusarium* species from SWO patients, they should analyze the affected nail for any signs of mixed variants or for infection emerging from beneath the proximal nail fold [1]. Gupta et al. highly recommended partitioned sampling in the presence of mixed variants, such as SWO and DLSO, and using it together with other diagnostic methods when appropriate. For infections involving both dermatophyte and non-dermatophyte molds, it is important to prioritize treatment of the dermatophyte and then subsequently treat any residual non-dermatophyte infection [8].

Treatment differs slightly for children due to their thin nail plates. Topical treatments are effective even when children have diffuse nail plate involvement, as their thin nails can facilitate drug penetration [7]. Although pediatric use of topical antifungals is not approved, topical amorolfine once a week has been reported as a successful treatment of SWO, due to *T. rubrum*, in an HIV-infected child. Adverse effects are unlikely, as this drug is not absorbed systemically [13].

Clinical Pearls for Reader

- Think of SWO in case of pseudo-leukonychia of the toenails.
- Keratin degranulation from continuous use of nail polish may mimic SWO.
- Think of molds in case of diffuse and deep involvement.
- Scrape the nail to distinguish between SWO originating from the proximal nail fold and PSO.
- Scraping of the affected nail and topical antifungal treat SWO in most cases.

References

1. Baran R, Faergemann J, Hay RJ. Superficial white onychomycosis–a syndrome with different fungal causes and paths of infection. J Am Acad Dermatol. 2007;57(5):879–82.
2. Almeida Jr HL, Boabaid RO, Timm V, Silva RM, Castro LA. Scanning electron microscopy of superficial white onychomycosis. An Bras Dermatol. 2015;90(5):753–5.
3. Baran R, Hay R, Perrin C. Superficial white onychomycosis revisited. J Eur Acad Dermatol Venereol. 2004;18(5):569–71.
4. Goodfield MJ, Evans EG. Treatment of superficial white onychomycosis with topical terbinafine cream. Br J Dermatol. 1999;141(3):604–5.
5. Hay RJ, Baran R. Onychomycosis: a proposed revision of the clinical classification. J Am Acad Dermatol. 2011;65(6):1219–27.
6. Baran R, Hay RJ, Tosti A, Haneke E. A new classification of onychomycosis. Br J Dermatol. 1998;139(4):567–71.

7. Piraccini BM, Tosti A. White superficial onychomycosis: epidemiological, clinical, and pathological study of 79 patients. Arch Dermatol. 2004;140(6):696–701.
8. Gupta AK, Summerbell RC. Combined distal and lateral subungual and white superficial onychomycosis in the toenails. J Am Acad Dermatol. 1999;41(6):938–44.
9. Effendy I, Lecha M, Feuilhade de Chauvin M, Di Chiacchio N, Baran R, European Onychomycosis Observatory. Epidemiology and clinical classification of onychomycosis. J Eur Acad Dermatol Venereol. 2005;19(Suppl 1):8–12.
10. Veer P, Patwardhan NS, Damle AS. Study of onychomycosis: prevailing fungi and pattern of infection. Indian J Med Microbiol. 2007;25(1):53–6.
11. Huang CC, Sun PL. Superficial white onychomycosis caused by Trichophyton verrucosum. Int J Dermatol. 2008;47(11):1162–4.
12. Walling HW, Sniezek PJ. Distribution of toenail dystrophy predicts histologic diagnosis of onychomycosis. J Am Acad Dermatol. 2007;56(6):945–8.
13. Pena-Penabad C, Garcia-Silva J, Almagro M, del Pozo J, Fonseca E. Superficial white onychomycosis in a 3-year-old human immunodeficiency virus-infected child. J Eur Acad Dermatol Venereol. 2001;15(1):51–3.

Chapter 5
Proximal Subungual Onychomycosis

George Glinos and Antonella Tosti

Key Features

- PSO can be caused by *dermatophytes*, *non-dermatophytic molds*, and *Candida* spp.
- PSO due to *dermatophytes* is rare.
- Most often seen in immunocompromised patients (e.g., AIDS, diabetes, transplant recipients).
- *T. rubrum* is the most common cause of infection.
- Infection starts at the proximal nail and progresses distally.

Introduction

Proximal subungual onychomycosis (PSO) is rare. In the traditional classification of this disease, the infection begins with fungal invasion of the proximal nail fold stratum corneum with subsequent infection of the matrix and deeper portions of the ventral nail plate [1–3]. From the proximal nail fold, fungi invade the proximal nail matrix and are incorporated into the newly forming nail, which accounts for the typically slow spread of PSO from the proximal nail fold to the fingertips (Fig. 5.1).

G. Glinos, BS
University of Miami Miller School of Medicine, Miami, FL, USA

A. Tosti, MD (✉)
Department of Dermatology and Cutaneous Surgery, University of Miami, Miami, FL 33136, USA
e-mail: atosti@med.miami.edu

A. Tosti et al. (eds.), *Onychomycosis*, DOI 10.1007/978-3-319-44853-4_5

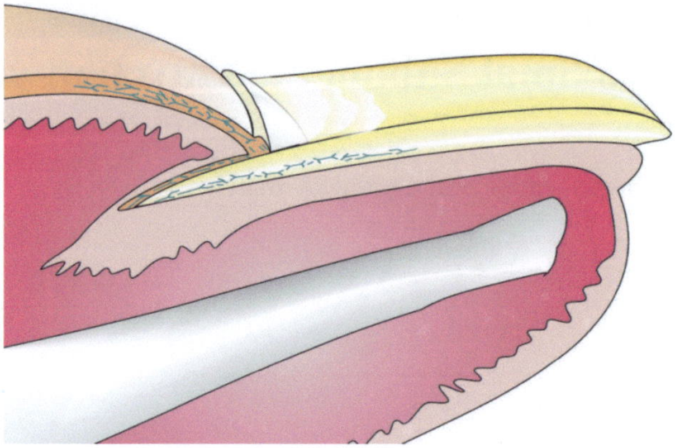

Fig. 5.1 Illustration of the classically described mechanism of pathogenesis in PSO. There is invasion of the proximal nail fold and nail matrix by fungi

Proximal nail plate invasion may occur secondary to acute or chronic paronychia, which is inflammation of the nail fold [4]. This route is most commonly seen with *Candida* [4].

More recently, alternative routes of infection have been described such as hematogenous spread and spread via the lymphatics, which can be exemplified by *maladie dermatophytique* [4, 5]. *Maladie dermatophytique* is a generalized dermatophytosis due to *T. schoenleinii* that affects the skin and internal organs alike [4]. Severe lymphadenopathy is observed in this condition, and biopsies of these enlarged lymph nodes have shown fungal hyphae, which is evidence of systemic spread of the fungal infection via lymphatics [5]. It is now thought that PSO can also be caused by fungal infection of the bloodstream; however, the exact mechanism of transfer from the blood to the nail plate is unclear [4]. Interestingly, there is some new evidence that PSO can progress from an isolated nail infection to a bloodstream infection, especially in immunosuppressed neutropenic patients [4]. The common link between all proposed mechanisms of infection is that fungi gain access to the proximal matrix that produces the ventral nail plate.

The most common organism causing PSO is *Trichophyton rubrum* [6], but many other dermatophytes have been identified such as *T. schoenleinii* [7], *T. megnini* [6, 8], *T. tonsurans* [6, 8], *T. mentagrophytes* [6], *T. epidermophyton* [6], *E. floccosum* [6], and *Microsporum sp.* [9]. Most cases are seen in immunocompromised individuals like HIV/AIDS [6, 8, 10], diabetics, dialysis, and transplant patients [7, 11]. PSO due to dermatophytes is not usually associated with periungual inflammation (Fig. 5.2). Some studies have noted that PSO occurs in up to one third of patients with serious or symptomatic HIV infection and can be considered a sign of immunodeficiency [12]. However, it is important to note that PSO in HIV patients has generally only been studied in those who have progressed to AIDS. Therefore, older data cannot be used to generalize PSO presentation or mycology in all

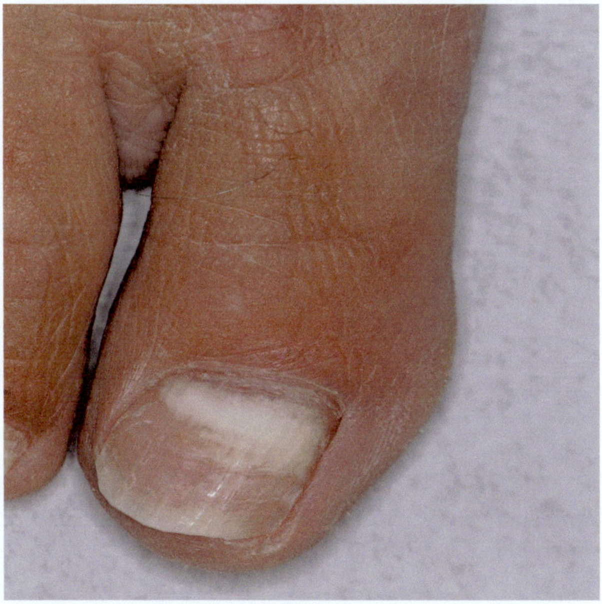

Fig. 5.2 PSO due to *T. rubrum* seen in an immunosuppressed patient

immunosuppressed patients, especially those with higher CD4 counts and without AIDS-defining complications. Moreover, most studies that investigated PSO in AIDS were conducted before the emergence of HAART, which is now the standard of care.

Several non-dermatophytic molds have been identified as causes of PSO including *Fusarium sp.* [13, 14], *Aspergillus fumigatus* [6, 15], *Aspergillus flavus* [16], *Scopulariopsis brevicaulis* [17], and *Acremonium sp.* [17]. Unlike PSO due to dermatophytes, these are not associated with immunosuppressed patients [17]. Non-dermatophytic molds are being increasingly considered a major cause of PSO in otherwise healthy patients. In the original classification of PSO, non-dermatophytic molds were thought to be contaminants, but further investigation has identified them as a significant cause of PSO. Of note, non-dermatophytic PSO is associated with significant periungual inflammation in many cases, which can help distinguish PSO due to dermatophytes from PSO due to non-dermatophytic molds clinically (Fig. 5.3). Distinguishing between dermatophytes and molds is important to guide treatment as their antifungal sensitivities are different.

Lastly, PSO can be caused by *Candida albicans* [6, 18]. *Candida* PSO is usually associated with paronychia, with the assumption that the inflammation can facilitate yeast invasion of the ventral nail plate. *Candida* PSO may rarely occur in chronic mucocutaneous candidiasis (CMCC) [18], a disorder of T cells that is characterized by chronic infection of mucosa, skin, and nails by *Candida*. In CCCA, *Candida* PSO is not always associated with paronychia and patients have a widespread

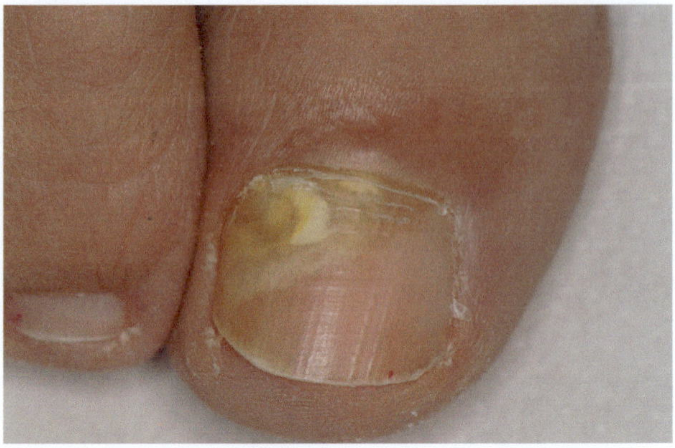

Fig. 5.3 PSO caused by a non-dermatophytic mold

mucocutaneous infection. Of note, the classic nail appearance in CMCC is granulomatous and totally dystrophic. Although PSO is not the most common nail presentation of CMCC, it can certainly be seen in this condition, and it has been reported in more recent literature [18].

Epidemiology

The exact prevalence of PSO is not clear due to a lack of large studies on the subject. Because it is most prevalent in immunocompromised patients, some studies have investigated PSO in this context. A study of onychomycosis in AIDS patients found that 55 of the 62 patients (88.7 %) who were seen for nail infections presented with PSO [6]. They also found that most (83 %) infections occurred in the feet [6]. Because these patients were immunosuppressed, the most common cause of infection were dermatophytes, with *T. rubrum* isolated in 36 (58 %) individuals followed by *T. mentagrophytes* (9.7 %) and *Epidermophyton floccosum* (4.8 %) [6]. Of note, some yeasts were isolated including *Candida albicans* (11.2 %) and *Pityrosporum ovale* (3.2 %) [6]. Of the non-dermatophytic molds, *S. brevicaulis* and *A. fumigatus* were isolated in four patients and one patient, respectively [6]. These non-dermatophytes were found coexisting with dermatophytes and never independently. Incorporating these results and other reports of PSO in the literature, PSO due to dermatophytes can be considered a sign of immunodeficiency [12].

Non-dermatophytic molds are another potential cause of PSO and are the most common cause of PSO in patients who are not immunosuppressed. Mold onychomycosis is not significantly associated with systemic diseases and should not be regarded as a sign of immunodeficiency as PSO due to dermatophytes is. A study at the University of Bologna [17] between 1995 and 1998 identified 59 patients out

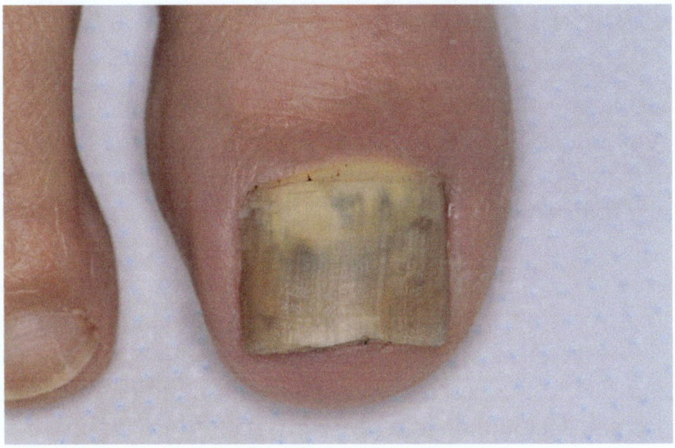

Fig. 5.4 PSO due to mold with associated periungual inflammation

of 1548 who were affected by onychomycosis due to non-dermatophytic molds. Molds were responsible for 13.6 % of all onychomycoses diagnosed via mycology culture, and the majority of these cases (76 %) presented with PSO. *Fusarium* sp. was identified in 44 % of these cases followed by 29 % *Scopulariopsis brevicaulis*, 15 % *Acremonium* sp., and 12 % *Aspergillus* sp. [17].

Furthermore, this study of non-dermatophytic molds identified an interesting relationship between molds and periungual inflammation. The researchers found that all cases of *Fusarium sp.* and *Aspergillus sp.*, as well as 59 % of cases of *S. brevicaulis*, were associated with significant periungual inflammation [17]. This contrasts to classic dermatophyte onychomycoses, which were found to almost never cause inflammation [17]. In fact, the authors noted that many of these patients with inflammation were initially treated with antibiotics and anti-inflammatory drugs due to their clinical presentation [17]. Thus, periungual inflammation is an important factor when developing a differential in PSO, and it may help influence what therapy the clinician will recommend (Fig. 5.4).

Generally speaking, the exact prevalence of certain fungi in PSO is unclear. In the past, PSO was thought to originate from periungual inflammation of the proximal nail fold. Also, it was commonly believed that non-dermatophytic molds that were isolated in cases of PSO were contaminants and not the cause of infection [17]. However, it has been revealed in more recent literature that PSO due to molds is frequently associated with periungual inflammation and that molds are a more common cause of PSO than was previously thought, which may invalidate much of our historical data. Furthermore, many of the studies analyzing PSO in the presence of HIV infection were conducted before HAART therapy became the standard of care. Many patients who were studied had extremely low CD4 counts, but today, clinicians can expect to see HIV patients with significantly lower degrees of immunosuppression due to HAART. Thus, one must be careful translating older data into modern clinical practice.

Clinical Features

Proximal subungual onychomycosis (PSO) is an infection of the ventral nail plate. It can be seen in both fingers and toes with the toes being more common. In the classic description of PSO, it begins with fungal invasion of the stratum corneum of proximal nail fold. There is subsequent infection of the deeper portions of the ventral nail plate, which is then followed by slow extension of the infection distally as the nail plate grows [1–3]. Eventually, the infection may involve the entire nail plate [1]. Clinically, this infection appears as a white leukonychia spreading distally as the nail plate grows. PSO causes true leukonychia as the white color is due to lack of light reflection due to the presence of fungi within the nail plate (Fig. 5.5). The nail surface is normal. The leukonychia can originate from the proximal nail fold or from the distal matrix with a single band that follows the shape of the lunula (Figs. 5.6 and 5.7).

Less commonly, the leukonychia can present as alternating transverse bands in which the infection spreads distally from the proximal nail fold in a similar way to the classic presentation, but the infection is remitting and relapsing, which gives the appearance of transverse bands of leukonychia separated by clinically and histologically normal nail plate (Fig. 5.8) [4, 18]. This intermittent dystrophy of the proximal

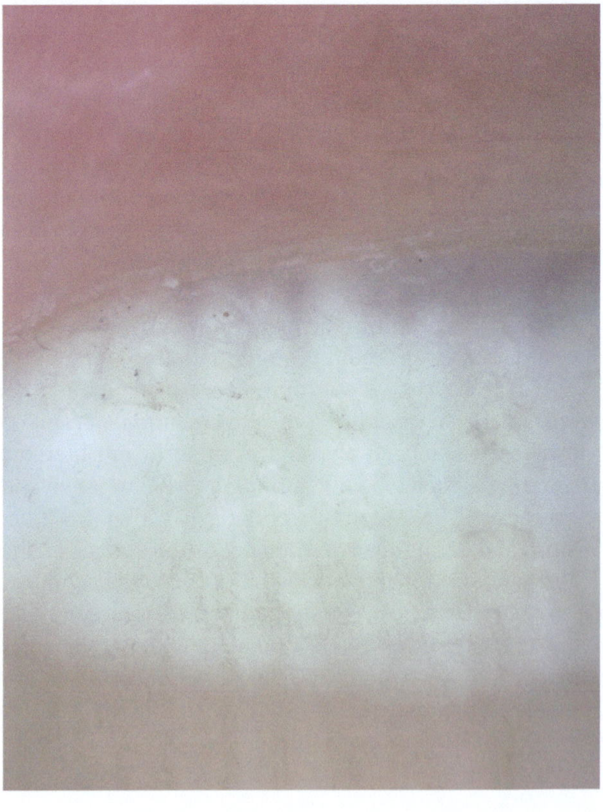

Fig. 5.5 Dermoscopy of PSO demonstrating true leukonychia. The nail surface is not affected, and the lack of light reflection is due to the presence of fungi within the nail plate

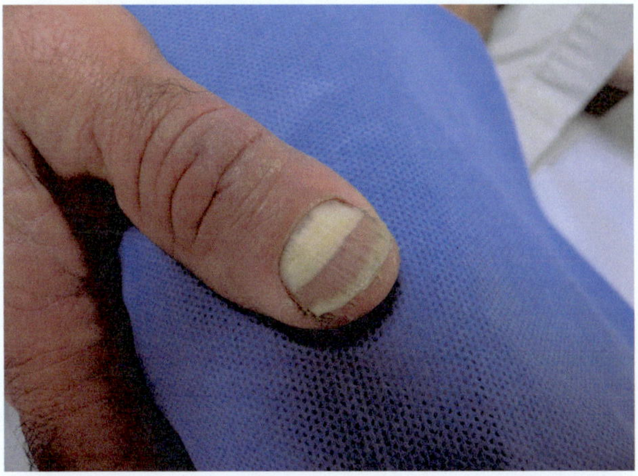

Fig. 5.6 Opaque *white* discoloration of the proximal nail in PSO

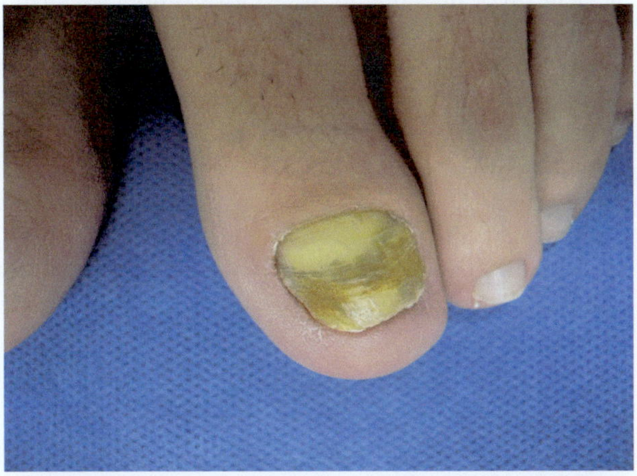

Fig. 5.7 PSO, the nail is dystrophic due to previous avulsions

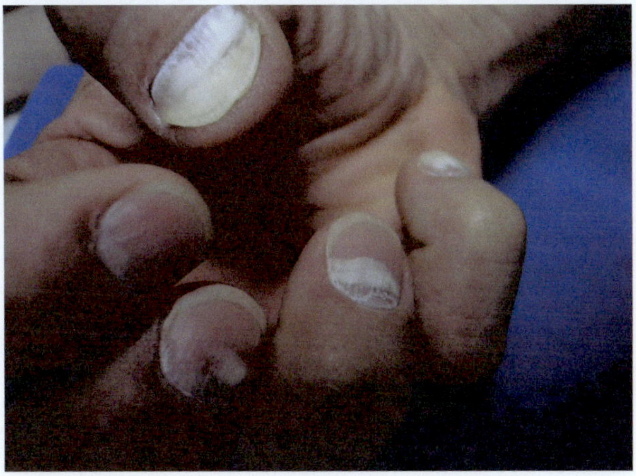

Fig. 5.8 PSO with alternating transverse bands as first described by Baran

nail plate will extend distally to give the appearance of transverse streaks of leukonychia like white waves, either single or multiple. These bands are not due to distal infection but rather proximal nail fold infection for two reasons. First, they have been followed at regular time intervals and are observed to extend distally from the proximal nail fold at a rate consistent with nail plate extension [18]. Second, the unique distal convexity of these transverse leukonychia lesions demonstrates that they are shaped by the lunula [18].

Although it is quite rare, PSO can be due to *Candida* infection. *Candida* usually causes a brownish discoloration of the nails along with severe onychodystrophy [18]. Its presentation can help differentiate it from other causes of PSO, which are mostly associated with white discoloration and milder onychodystrophy. *Candida* PSO is classically seen in those with paronychia and is thought to occur because the inflammation can facilitate yeast invasion to the ventral nail plate. It has also been reported in patients with chronic mucocutaneous candidiasis (CMCC) [18]. In CMCC, PSO due to *Candida* is not always associated with paronychia, and the mechanism of infection in these cases is not clear. Thus, it is important to maintain a high level of suspicion for *Candida* when patients have PSO associated with paronychia but also to appreciate that paronychia is not a defining factor, especially if the patient presents with other mucocutaneous findings.

In regards to symptomatology, patients with PSO may range from being asymptomatic to experiencing pain or discomfort to the degree that it interferes with walking or standing. In PSO due to non-dermatophytic molds, periungual inflammation is especially common and may be quite painful with surrounding erythema and edema. Some cases may even be associated with purulent discharge, which tends to cause these patients to be frequently misdiagnosed as having a bacterial infection.

Diagnostic Clues

PSO should always be considered in the differential diagnosis of true leukonychia.

Diagnosis of fungal infection can be made by visualization of fungal hyphae or fungal elements under direct light microscopy of 20 % potassium hydroxide (KOH) preparation in dimethyl sulfoxide (DMSO). This is the fastest and least expensive option; however, in the case of PSO, it can be challenging to obtain a sample. First, the target site should be cleaned with ethanol to prevent contamination [19]. One must pare the nail plate with a blade to access the ventral side, scraping the white portions of the nail plate, and preparation with KOH will usually reveal abundant hyphal elements under the microscope [1]. Newer techniques such as vertical drilling, horizontal drilling, or subungual curettage have emerged as viable options to obtain samples [20].

The authors like to utilize 3 mm punch to take a big sample that can be divided and utilized for KOH preparation, cultures, and pathology (Fig. 5.9).

Once a sample is obtained, mycological culture should be conducted in addition to other tests using Sabouraud dextrose agar [19]. Littman Oxgall, Borelli medium,

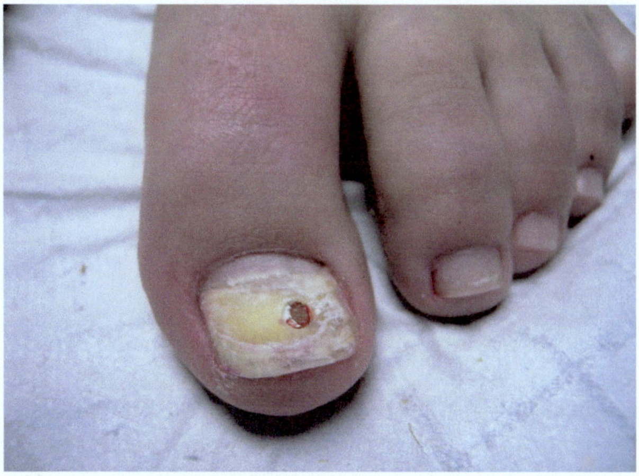

Fig. 5.9 Sample can be taken with a 3 mm punch biopsy for histopathological analysis

or potato dextrose agar may also be used. The samples must be incubated at 26–30 ° C for several weeks to 1 month. It is important to select agar without cycloheximide, which is a common additive. Cycloheximide is added to inhibit the growth of non-dermatophytic molds, but we now know these are an important cause of PSO [19]. When a mold is suspected, it is recommended to serially sample the patient's nails at different points of time to confirm the repeated presence of non-dermatophytic mold to ensure that the non-dermatophytic mold is part of the primary infection and not a contaminant [19]. Fungi are notoriously difficult to culture. Not only does this method of diagnosis take a long time, but sensitivity and specificity is limited by fungal viability on the chosen medium as well as sampling technique.

On histopathology, nail samples are stained with periodic acid-Schiff (PAS) or grocott's methenamine silver (GMS). With the PAS technique, the fungi are stained magenta, but it only works on living fungi. With the GMS technique, the fungi are stained dark brown on a background of pale green, and it works for both living and dead fungi. As with other techniques, it is key to identify fungi in the ventral nail plate. This method has high sensitivity and specificity, especially in the hands of an experienced histopathologist.

In the current literature, several studies have investigated the applicability of these various diagnostic techniques. Generally, histopathological examination with PAS staining (HPE-PAS) is found to have the highest positive predictive value and negative predictive value and is regarded as the gold standard for diagnosis of onychomycosis [21, 22]. However, not many studies have focused on comparing diagnostic methods in PSO specifically. It can be assumed that these diagnostic tests may have similar predictive value in PSO, but that cannot be known with certainty at this time.

Lastly, newer PCR techniques have been introduced for the diagnosis of onychomycoses and offer some advantages over traditional diagnostic methods [23]. PCR provides a much faster diagnosis within days versus weeks with traditional culture. Also, it has less vulnerable errors due to contamination, fungal viability, or sampling technique [23].

The key to making any diagnosis of PSO is to sample the ventral nail plate. Diagnosis may be difficult due to its atypical clinical presentation, but always maintain an appropriate level of suspicion when a patient displays one of the presentations noted earlier in this chapter.

Summary for the Clinician

Proximal subungual onychomycosis (PSO) is an infection of the proximal ventral nail plate. It can be due to dermatophytes, non-dermatophytic molds, or *Candida*. PSO due to dermatophytes is rare and is most frequently found in patients with suppressed immune systems, especially HIV/AIDS, or in patients taking systemic immunosuppressors. The most common agent in these cases is *Trichophyton rubrum*, but other dermatophytes have also been implicated. Non-dermatophytic molds have emerged as a more common cause of PSO than previously thought. These cases are not associated with immunosuppression and are often associated with significant periungual inflammation. Less commonly, yeasts like *Candida* can be the causal pathogen. Classically, PSO is seen as a white patch in proximal nail plate and extending distally as the nail grows; however, other less common presentations like alternating transverse bands have been described. It can be diagnosed by KOH prep microscopy, histopathologic analysis, culture, and PCR. Obtaining an adequate sample of the ventral nail plate is key to diagnosis.

Clinical Pearls

- Maintain a high level of suspicion for PSO in immunosuppressed patients with proximal nail leukonychia.
- Think of molds in case of PSO associated with periungual inflammation.
- A 3 mm punch can be utilized to obtain a sample from the ventral nail plate.
- PSO requires systemic treatment.

References

1. Zaias N. Onychomycosis. Arch Dermatol. 1972;105(2):263–74.
2. Zaias N. Onychomycosis. Dermatol Clin. 1985;3(3):445–60.
3. Weinberg JM, Koestenblatt EK, Don PC, White SM, Stein MN, Bamji M. Proximal white subungual onychomycosis in the immunocompetent patient: report of two cases and review of the literature. Acta Derm Venereol. 1999;79(1):81–2.
4. Hay RJ, Baran R. Onychomycosis: a proposed revision of the clinical classification. J Am Acad Dermatol. 2011;65(6):1219–27.

5. Baran R, Mcloone N, Hay RJ. Could proximal white subungual onychomycosis be a complication of systemic spread? The lessons to be learned from Maladie Dermatophytique and other deep infections. Br J Dermatol. 2005;153(5):1023–5.
6. Dompmartin D, Dompmartin A, Deluol AM, Grosshans E, Coulaud JP. Onychomycosis and AIDS. Clinical and laboratory findings in 62 patients. Int J Dermatol. 1990;29(5):337–9.
7. Chang P, Arenas R. Proximal white subungual onychomycosis in a kidney transplant patient. Int J Dermatol. 1995;34(8):591.
8. Silva-Lizama E, Logemann H. Proximal white subungual onychomycosis in AIDS. Int J Dermatol. 1996;35(4):290–1.
9. Piraccini BM, Morelli R, Stinchi C, Tosti A. Proximal subungual onychomycosis due to Microsporum canis. Br J Dermatol. 1996;134(1):175–7.
10. Noppakun N, Head ES. Proximal white subungual onychomycosis in a patient with acquired immune deficiency syndrome. Int J Dermatol. 1986;25(9):586–7.
11. Lee MM, Diven DG, Smith EB, Pupo RA. Onychomycosis. Arch Dermatol. 1990;126(3):402.
12. Rongioletti F, Persi A, Tripodi S, Rebora A. Proximal white subungual onychomycosis: a sign of immunodeficiency. J Am Acad Dermatol. 1994;30(1):129–30.
13. Baran R, Tosti A, Piraccini BM. Uncommon clinical patterns of Fusarium nail infection: report of three cases. Br J Dermatol. 1997;136(3):424–7.
14. Ranawaka RR, Nagahawatte A, Gunasekara TA. Fusarium onychomycosis: prevalence, clinical presentations, response to itraconazole and terbinafine pulse therapy, and 1-year follow-up in nine cases. Int J Dermatol. 2015;54(11):1275–82.
15. Tosti A, Piraccini BM. Proximal subungual onychomycosis due to Aspergillus niger: report of two cases. Br J Dermatol. 1998;139(1):156–7.
16. Choudhary SV, Koley S, Mallick S, Bose S, Basak S. Proximal subungual onychomycosis caused by Aspergillus flavus in a HIV-positive patient. Indian J Dermatol Venereol Leprol. 2009;75(4):410–2.
17. Tosti A, Piraccini BM, Lorenzi S. Onychomycosis caused by nondermatophytic molds: clinical features and response to treatment of 59 cases. J Am Acad Dermatol. 2000;42(2 Pt 1):217–24.
18. Baran R. Proximal subungual Candida onychomycosis. An unusual manifestation of chronic mucocutaneous candidiasis. Br J Dermatol. 1997;137(2):286–8.
19. Gupta AK, Simpson FC. Diagnosing onychomycosis. Clin Dermatol. 2013;31(5):540–3.
20. Shemer A, Davidovici B, Grunwald MH, Trau H, Amichai B. Comparative study of nail sampling techniques in onychomycosis. J Dermatol. 2009;36(7):410–4.
21. Weinberg JM, Koestenblatt EK, Tutrone WD, Tishler HR, Najarian L. Comparison of diagnostic methods in the evaluation of onychomycosis. J Am Acad Dermatol. 2003;49(2):193–7.
22. Jeelani S, Ahmed QM, Lanker AM, Hassan I, Jeelani N, Fazili T. Histopathological examination of nail clippings using PAS staining (HPE-PAS): gold standard in diagnosis of Onychomycosis. Mycoses. 2015;58(1):27–32.
23. Rosen T, Friedlander SF, Kircik L, et al. Onychomycosis: epidemiology, diagnosis, and treatment in a changing landscape. J Drugs Dermatol. 2015;14(3):223–33.

Chapter 6
Endonyx Onychomycosis

Vidhi V. Shah and Antonella Tosti

Key Feature Box

- Endonyx onychomycosis is a fungal infection of the nails caused by *Trichophyton soudanense*, *Trichophyton violaceum*, and *Trichophyton rubrum*.
- Patients with endonyx onychomycosis present with milky-white discoloration of the nail plate without hyperkeratosis or onycholysis.
- Histopathology will demonstrate an abundance of fungal filaments confined to the nail plate without nail bed inflammation or hyphae.
- Treatment typically consists of oral and topical antifungal therapies; however, recalcitrant infections may necessitate combination therapy, chemical and/or surgical plate avulsion, or photodynamic therapy.

Introduction

Endonyx onychomycosis (EO) is an exceedingly rare pattern of fungal infection of the nail plate associated with the endothrix dermatophytes *Trichophyton soudanense*, *Trichophyton violaceum*, and *Trichophyton rubrum* [1–4]. Currently, there is only one report in the literature of endonyx onychomycosis caused by *Trichophyton tonsurans* [5]. In endonyx, fungal hyphae infect and directly invade the superficial and deep portions of the nail plate [4]. This unique pattern of nail invasion is conceivably related to these organisms' high affinity for hard keratins [4].

V.V. Shah, BA • A. Tosti, MD (✉)
Department of Dermatology and Cutaneous Surgery, University of Miami, Miami, FL, USA
e-mail: shahvidhiv@gmail.com; atosti@med.miami.edu

A. Tosti et al. (eds.), *Onychomycosis*, DOI 10.1007/978-3-319-44853-4_6

Epidemiology

Endonyx onychomycosis appears to affect both men and women equally and is found among all age groups and ethnicities [1, 2, 6]. The exact incidence of this nail infection remains unknown; however, it is likely to be more prevalent in areas where *Trichophyton* species is endemic, such as in central and west Africa [2].

Clinical Features

Endonyx onychomycosis is clinically characterized a milky-white discoloration of the nail plate. The nail plate surface is normal and the nail has a normal thickness [3, 4]. The nail plate will be firmly attached to the nail bed [4]. The absence of hyperkeratosis and onycholysis separates endonyx from other entities, such as distal subungual onychomycosis [4]. Table 6.1 illustrates clinical features commonly present and absent in endonyx onychomycosis.

Diagnostic Clues

Endonyx onychomycosis should be distinguished from proximal subungual onychomycosis as both present with white nail discoloration without onycholysis or subungual hyperkeratosis. History and clinical examination can help in differential diagnosis. In EO invasion occurs from distal margin, and nail discoloration starts distally and progresses proximally (Fig. 6.1) in contrast with proximal subungual onychomycosis (PSO) that originates proximally and progresses distally.

Diagnosis of endonyx onychomycosis should be confirmed by direct microscopic examination and fungal cultures. Periodic acid-Schiff (PAS) stain will demonstrate tunnels of fungal elements arranged either longitudinally or transversely within the entire thickness of the nail plate [4, 6]. Importantly, there are no signs of fungal invasion or inflammation in the nail bed [4]. Culture of the nail clippings will expose the causative organism [6].

Table 6.1 Present and absent clinical features in endonyx onychomycosis

Present features	Absent features
Normal nail plate surface	Superficial desquamation
Normal nail plate thickness	Hyperkeratosis
Nail plate firmly attached to the nail bed	Onycholysis
Milky-white nail plate discoloration	Subungual changes
Nail plate fungal hyphae	Periungual inflammation

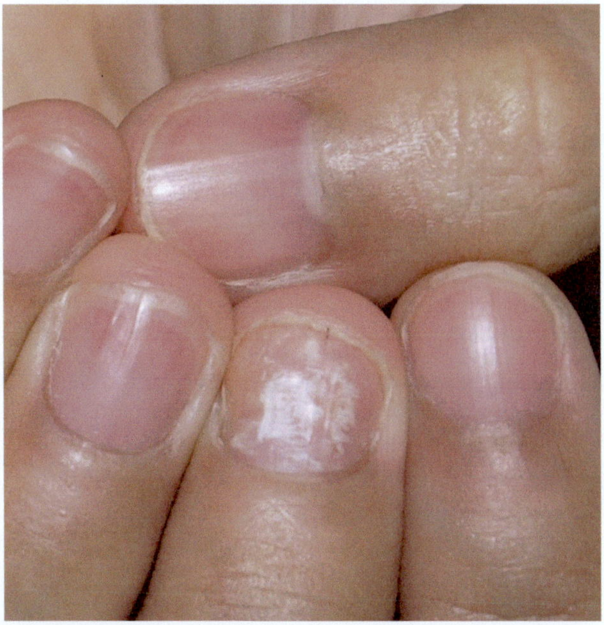

Fig. 6.1 Endonyx onychomycosis of the fingernail. The nail plate shows distal leukonychia in the absence of subungual hyperkeratosis (Courtesy of Chinmanat Tangjaturonrusamee MD)

Summary for the Clinician

Endonyx is a rare form of onychomycosis that affects all ages and both genders. Clinicians should be aware of the presentation of this rare entity, as certain forms may be resistant to standard antifungal therapy [6]. The presence of milky-white discoloration of the nail plate in the absence of hyperkeratosis and onycholysis suggests endonyx pattern [4]. PAS staining for fungal elements confined to the nail plate may help validate the diagnosis [4]. Consider treatment with standard topical and oral antifungals first, followed by combination therapy, chemical and/or surgical plate avulsion, or photodynamic therapy if the infection is difficult to treat.

Clinical Pearls

- Endonyx is an unusual variant of onychomycosis that affects men and women of all ages, races, and ethnicities.
- Patients present with opaque-white discoloration of the nail plate without subungual changes.
- Superficial nail plate involvement, hyperkeratosis, onycholysis, or nail bed inflammation should prompt consideration of an alternative diagnosis.
- Direct microscopic examination with PAS staining that demonstrates plenty of fungal hyphae in the nail plate, but none in the nail bed, is pathognomonic of endonyx.

References

1. Souza LW, Souza SV, Botelho AC. Endonyx toenail onychomycosis caused by Trichophyton rubrum: treatment with photodynamic therapy based on methylene blue dye. An Bras Dermatol. 2013;88(6):1019–21. doi:10.1590/abd1806-4841.20132180.
2. Fletcher CL, Moore MK, Hay RJ. Endonyx onychomycosis due to Trichophyton soudanense in two Somalian siblings. Br J Dermatol. 2001;145(4):687–8.
3. Hay RJ, Baran R. Onychomycosis: a proposed revision of the clinical classification. J Am Acad Dermatol. 2011;65(6):1219–27. doi:10.1016/j.jaad.2010.09.730.
4. Tosti A, Baran R, Piraccini BM, Fanti PA. "Endonyx" onychomycosis: a new modality of nail invasion by dermatophytes. Acta Derm Venereol. 1999;79(1):52–3.
5. Bunyaratavej S, Bunyaratavej S, Muanprasart C, Matthapan L, Varothai S, Tangjaturonrusamee C, et al. Endonyx onychomycosis caused by Trichophyton tonsurans. Indian J Dermatol Venereol Leprol. 2015;81(4):390–2. doi:10.4103/0378-6323.157460.
6. Mulvaney PM, Telang GH, Jellinek N. Trichophytum rubrum endonyx onychomycosis resistant to standard oral and topical therapies. Dermatol Online J. 2015;21(9).

Chapter 7
Onychomycoses Due to Non-dermatophytic Molds

Austin J. Maddy, Jennifer L. Abrahams, and Antonella Tosti

Key Features

- Non-dermatophytic molds have been increasingly recognized as agents of onychomycosis.
- Prevalence of non-dermatophytic onychomycosis depends on geographic areas.
- Molds can cause different types of onychomycosis including proximal subungual, "deep" white superficial, and distal subungual onychomycosis.
- Diagnosis of mold onychomycosis is more complex than the dermatophytic counterpart and requires microscopic examination and culture on multiple samples.
- Treatment is difficult and often requires combination of topical antifungals, systemic antifungals, and chemical avulsion.

Introduction

Non-dermatophytic molds are filamentous fungi that are regularly found in nature as soil saprophytes and plant pathogens. Molds can frequently colonize the nails and be isolated in cultures without having a pathologic significance. However, molds can also invade the nails and cause onychomycosis, and prevalence of mold infections has been increasing worldwide in the last several decades. Diagnosis of mold onychomycosis requires a strict correlation between nail abnormalities and mycologic findings as well as isolation of the same organism from multiple samples and inoculates. Concomitant infections with molds and dermatophytes can also occur.

A.J. Maddy • J.L. Abrahams, MD • A. Tosti (✉)
Department of Dermatology and Cutaneous Surgery, University of Miami Miller School of Medicine, Miami, FL, USA
e-mail: atosti@med.miami.edu

A. Tosti et al. (eds.), *Onychomycosis*, DOI 10.1007/978-3-319-44853-4_7

Molds that can cause onychomycosis include but are not limited to *Scopulariopsis brevicaulis*, *Aspergillus* spp., *Acremonium* spp., *Alternaria* spp., *Chrysosporium* spp., *Aureobasidium pullulans*, *Curvularia* spp., *Penicillium* spp., *Fusarium* spp., *Onychocola canadensis*, *Exophiala* spp., *Ulocladium* spp., *Nattrassia mangiferae*, and *Neoscytalidium dimidiatum* [1, 3, 7, 14, 17–19, 33, 42].

Prevalence of mold onychomycosis varies in different countries depending on geographic area, climate, and lifestyle conditions [4]. Incidence of the infection increases with age, with most patients being older than 40 years [1, 4, 6, 8, 18, 42].

Treatment of mold onychomycosis is even more difficult than dermatophytic onychomycosis. Combination of topical antifungals, chemical nail avulsion, and systemic antifungals is often required.

Epidemiology

Approximately 10 % of onychomycoses are caused by non-dermatophytic molds [2, 5, 14]. Frequencies as high as 22 % [30], 45.8 % [17], 51.6 % [36], and even 68 % [44] have been reported in various countries. Data in the United States is limited since most doctors do not take a culture sample (Table 7.1).

Most cases of mold onychomycosis are caused by *Scopulariopsis brevicaulis* [3, 11, 20, 37, 38, 40, 43] or *Aspergillus* spp. [4, 18, 30, 41, 42, 44]. Most infections of non-dermatophytic molds are found in the hot and humid tropical and subtropical parts of the world [3, 21, 30]. Prevalence varies globally, depending on the climate and microenvironment of each geographic region. *Acremonium* spp., *Aspergillus* spp., and *Neoscytalidium* spp. are common in Canada [32]. *Fusarium* spp., *Acremonium* spp., and *Scopulariopsis brevicaulis* are common in the United States [45]. *Neoscytalidium* spp. and *Fusarium* spp. are found throughout South America (especially prevalent in Colombia and Brazil) [33, 35]. *Scopulariopsis brevicaulis*, *Aspergillus* spp., and *Fusarium* spp. are frequently isolated in Pakistan [36]. *Neoscytalidium dimidiatum* and *Fusarium* spp. are found in Thailand [36], while *Scopulariopsis brevicaulis*, *Aspergillus* spp., *Acremonium* spp., and *Fusarium* spp. are common in the Mediterranean (Italy, Greece, and Turkey) [37–39, 42].

The most important predisposing factor is, as for dermatophytes, patient's age. Studies of non-dermatophytic mold onychomycosis report most afflicted patients being older than 40 years [1, 4, 6, 8, 18, 43]. Possible reasons include slower nail growth rate with aging, repeated nail trauma, prolonged exposure to pathogenic fungi, and venous insufficiency. Toenails are generally more often affected than fingernails, due to their slower growth rate.

Onychomycosis from non-dermatophytic molds is more common in females, in contrast to dermatophytic onychomycosis [1, 31, 32]. In a Colombian study of 310 cases of non-dermatophytic mold onychomycosis with toenail infections, women represented 62 % of cases [31].

Table 7.1 Percentage of non-dermatophytic mold onychomycosis due to mold pathogens in different countries

	United States [45]	Canada [32]	Iran [41]	Brazil [33]	Colombia [34]	Pakistan [35]	Thailand [36]	Italy [37]	Greece [38]	India [4]	Turkey [42]
Total percentage of onychomycosis due to NDM	20.7 %	4.3 %	11.5 %	7.4 %	14 %	11 %	51.6 %	9 %	15.5 %	35.3 %	9 %
Scopulariopsis brevicaulis	20.5 %	–	2.1 %	–	–	18.2 %	–	35.3 %	65.9 %	3.8 %	3 %
Aspergillus species	11.4 %	33 %	59.6 %	8.1 %	–	18.2 %	–	27.5 %	4.5 %	85 %	22 %
Acremonium species	29.5 %	33 %	17 %	–	–	9.1 %	–	5.9 %	22.8 %	–	18 %
Neoscytalidium species	4.5 %	17 %	–	–	38 %	9.1 %	70.6 %	–	–	–	–
Fusarium species	34.1 %	–	12.7 %	60.8 %	42.9 %	36.4 %	29.4 %	27.5 %	–	3.8 %	18 %
Nattrassia mangiferae	–	–	–	31.1 %	–	–	–	–	–	–	–
Alternaria species	–	–	–	–	–	9.1 %	–	–	4.5 %	–	3 %
Ulocladium species	–	–	–	–	–	–	–	–	–	–	12 %

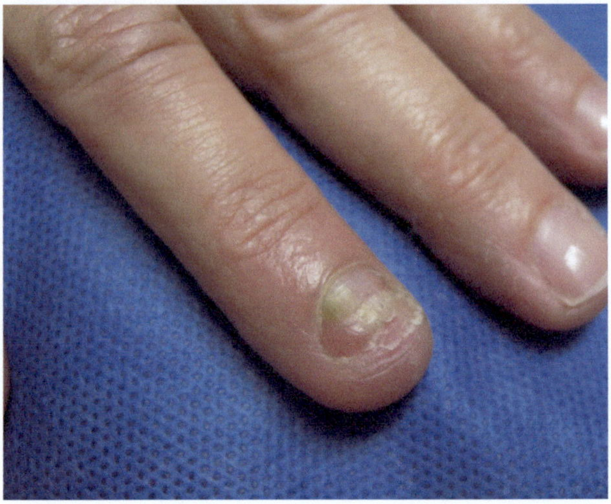

Fig. 7.1 Proximal subungual onychomycosis with periungual inflammation due to *Fusarium* spp.

Clinical Features

Non-dermatophytic molds can cause proximal subungual, “deep” white superficial, and distal subungual onychomycosis.

Proximal subungual onychomycosis is characterized by the invasion of the nail matrix through the proximal nail folds. Fungi are then incorporated in the ventral nail plate from the matrix. The proximal nail plate shows a yellow-white discoloration as presence of fungal elements changes nail plate transparency. Presence of erythema and swelling of proximal and lateral nail folds is common (Fig. 7.1). Inflammation can be prominent in some cases and purulent discharge might occur. Proximal subungual onychomycosis is commonly associated with the following molds: *Fusarium* spp., *Aspergillus* spp., and *Scopulariopsis brevica*ulis [24]. *Fusarium* and *Scopulariopsis brevicaulis* produce a yellow-white discoloration of the proximal nail plate [23, 24], while *Aspergillus* can be associated with a black or green discoloration [25, 26]. The presence of periungual inflammation strongly suggests a mold infection, as this feature is almost never seen in proximal subungual onychomycosis caused by dermatophytes (Fig. 7.2) [5].

Deep white superficial onychomycosis is characterized by opaque, friable, white, superficial lesions that start on the dorsal surface of the nail plate, usually on the toes [26]. Mold infections differ from classic white superficial onychomycosis caused by dermatophytes because the infection is deeper and more diffuse (Fig. 7.3a, b) [27, 29]. Deep white superficial onychomycosis is commonly seen with *Fusarium* spp., *Acremonium* spp., and *Aspergillus* spp. [22, 27, 28].

Distal subungual onychomycosis is primarily a nail bed disorder. Infection usually begins with involvement of the distal part of the nail bed and progresses proximally along the ventral surface of the nail plate. It most commonly affects the great

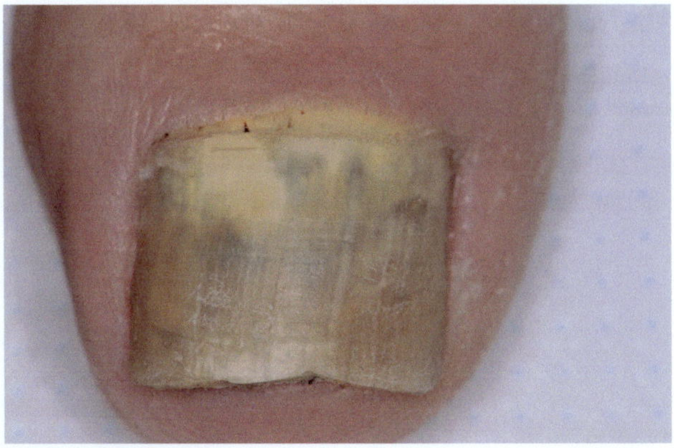

Fig. 7.2 Proximal subungual onychomycosis with periungual inflammation due to *Aspergillus* spp.

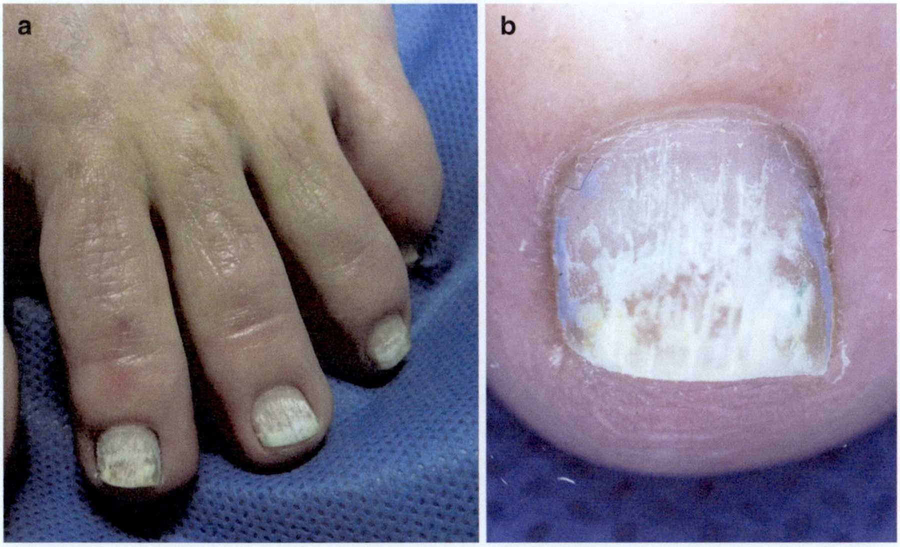

Fig. 7.3 (**a**, **b**) Deep white superficial onychomycosis (**a**) dermoscopy shows invasion of the intermediate nail plate (**b**)

toe [7]. The nails become thick due to subungual hyperkeratosis, which is associated with onycholysis. The onycholytic nail plate is yellowish white to brown in color (Fig. 7.4). Agents responsible for distal subungual onychomycosis include *Acremonium* spp., *Fusarium* spp., and *Alternaria* spp. [5, 7, 8]. Periungual inflammation may be seen in distal subungual onychomycosis caused by *Fusarium* spp. [5]. Tinea pedis is not commonly associated with mold onychomycosis, although it can be seen in *Scopulariopsis brevicaulis* infections.

Pigmented onychomycosis is characterized by a brown or black discoloration of the nail plate due to melanin deposition (Fig. 7.5a, b). Non-dermatophytic molds

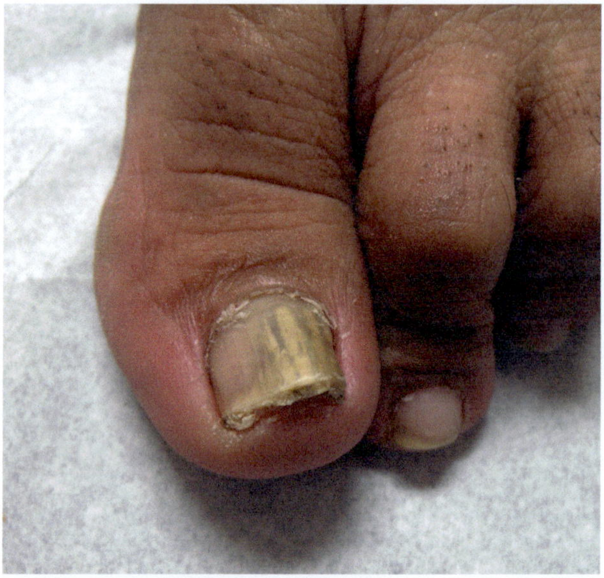

Fig. 7.4 Distal subungual onychomycosis from molds

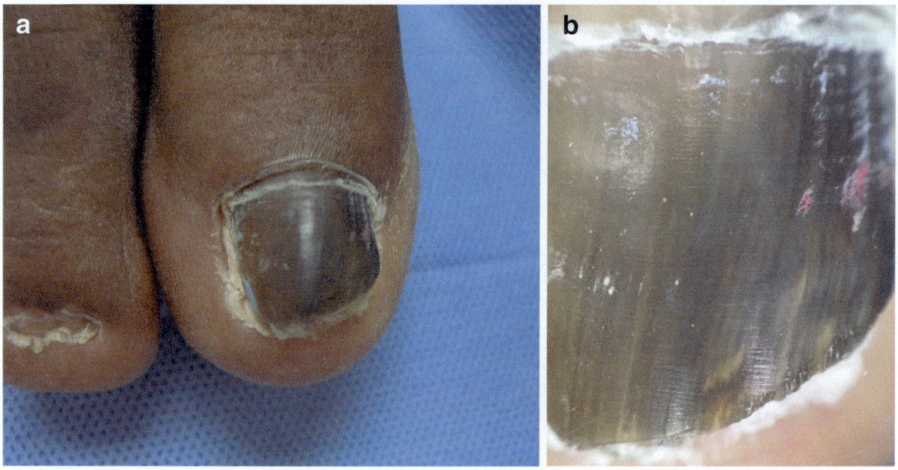

Fig. 7.5 (**a**, **b**) Pigmented distal subungual onychomycosis (**a**) dermoscopy shows yellow-white striae that suggest diagnosis (**b**)

causing pigmented onychomycosis include the dematiaceous fungi *Neoscytalidium dimidiatum*, *Alternaria* spp., and *Exophiala* spp. [7]. These organisms produce melanin, which is incorporated into their cell walls or secreted extracellularly, causing them to appear brown or black when cultured. Pigmented onychomycosis can diffusely affect the entire nail or present as a longitudinal band, mimicking a pigmented lesion (Fig. 7.6) [9]. *Neoscytalidium dimidiatum* can also cause tinea manuum and tinea pedis.

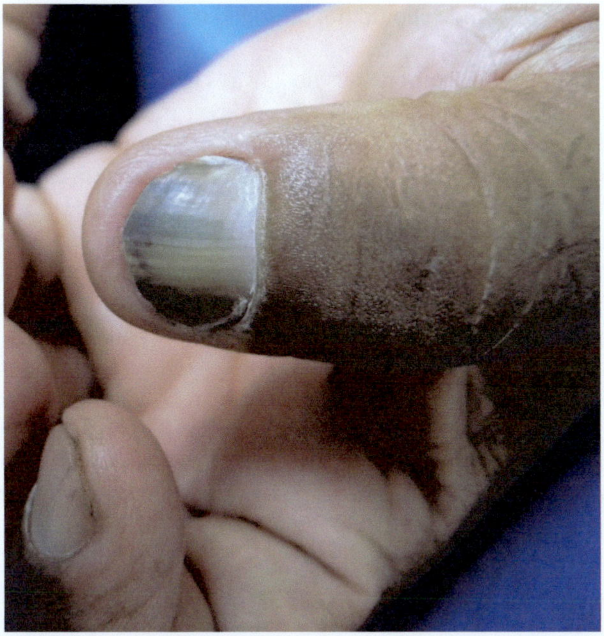

Fig. 7.6 Pigmented onychomycosis mimicking a pigmented lesion

Diagnosis

Nail collection techniques for mycological examination vary depending on the clinical presentation of the mold onychomycosis. In proximal subungual onychomycosis, samples should be obtained from the deep ventral nail plate. This can be easily done using a 3 mm punch or drilling the nail with a scalpel blade. In white superficial onychomycosis, samples are obtained by scraping the affected nail surface [6]. In cases of distal subungual onychomycosis, the sample should include subungual debris from the more proximal part of the lesion. It is very important to alert the lab about possibility of mold infection as dermatophytic media contain factors that inhibit mold growth.

If the physician suspects an infection due to a non-dermatophytic mold, a specimen should be obtained and sent to the mycology lab for confirmatory culture. Pathology of nail clippings does not distinguish between molds and dermatophytes and is not diagnostic in cases of mold infections [10]. Fungal culture mediums generally contain Sabouraud dextrose agar (SDA), along with antibiotics such as gentamicin and chloramphenicol [10, 19] to deter competitive bacterial growth. Non-dermatophytic molds grow faster than dermatophytes and are typically viewed as contaminants in the lab and will grow in SDA along with dermatophytes and yeasts. Cycloheximide is routinely added to the SDA medium in order to inhibit growth of the molds. If a non-dermatophytic mold is suspected, the lab must be informed that cycloheximide should not be added in order to allow for mold growth and isolation.

Direct microscopic observation does not always result in a positive diagnosis, and one study has shown that more than 42 % of direct microscopic exams were false negatives [1]. Mycologic diagnosis of mold infection requires strict criteria as molds can be common contaminants. The following is considered as "gold standard": microscopic observation of hyphae and/or conidia in 10 % KOH preparations, isolation of the same non-dermatophytic mold in at least three inoculates in two repeated samplings, and failure to isolate a dermatophyte. If a dermatophyte is isolated by culture, there is immediate pathogenic confirmation, unlike the necessary repeated inoculates required to confirm non-dermatophytic mold pathogenesis.

Polymerase chain reaction (PCR) can amplify small fragments of DNA from a fungal biopsy for identification. Fungal species can be identified from the original sample through quantitative PCR, sequencing of PCR amplification products, or restriction fragment length polymorphism digestion analysis [12]. Advantages of PCR include the rapidity and sensitivity, but its use is still limited even though costs are becoming very competitive. This technique cannot distinguish contaminants from pathogens.

Treatment

Treatments of onychomycosis due to non-dermatophytic molds include topical antifungals, systemic antifungals, and chemical nail avulsion.

Non-dermatophytic molds generally do not respond well to systemic therapy, although this is not an absolute. For example, *Fusarium* spp., *Acremonium* spp., *Neoscytalidium* spp., and *Scopulariopsis brevicaulis* rarely respond to systemic medications [23], while *Aspergillus* spp. is sensitive to systemics [5]. Systemic therapy can be given with itraconazole, terbinafine, or fluconazole (not FDA approved for this indication). At times, combinations of systemic, topical, and avulsion treatments may provide the best outcomes for the patient. When systemic therapy is contraindicated, topical agents and/or chemical and surgical avulsion may be used.

Photodynamic therapy (PDT) with topical 5-aminolevulinic acid (ALA) or methyl aminolevulinate (MAL) [16] is another treatment modality for distal subungual onychomycosis due to molds. For PDT to be effective against onychomycosis, it is important to remove the nail plate as the photosensitizers need to reach the affected nail bed [13]. This can be achieved using urea ointment [12]. PDT has been established as an effective treatment of non-dermatophytic molds including *Acremonium sclerotigenum* [15].

Summary for the Clinician

- It is important to consider non-dermatophytic molds as causative agents of onychomycosis as rates of infections with these pathogenic agents are increasing.
- Diagnosis of mold infection can only be done by culture or PCR, as fungal stains of nail clippings do not provide discriminatory identification.
- Mold onychomycosis should always be considered in patients presenting with proximal subungual onychomycosis with periungual inflammation, deep white superficial onychomycosis, and pigmented onychomycosis.

Clinical Pearls for the Reader

- Think of molds in cases of proximal subungual onychomycosis associated with erythema and swelling of the proximal/lateral nail folds.
- Think of molds in cases of white superficial onychomycosis that diffusely affect the nail and cannot easily be scraped away.
- Think of molds in cases of pigmented onychomycosis.
- Tinea pedis is not common in association with mold onychomycosis.
- Inform the lab when submitting culture specimens in which you suspect a pathogenic mold.
- Combination of systemic, topical, and podiatric treatments is often required.

References

1. Bombace F, Iovene MR, Galdiero M, Martora F, Nicoletti GF, D'Andrea M, Della Pepa ME, Vitiello M. Non-dermatophytic onychomycosis diagnostic criteria: an unresolved question. Mycoses. 2016; doi:10.1111/myc.12504.
2. Welsh O, Vera-Cabrera L, Welsh E. Onychomycosis. Clin Dermatol. 2010;28:151–9.
3. Velez A, Linares Ma J, Fenandez-Roldan JC, Casal M. Study of onychomycosis in Cordoba, Spain: prevailing fungi and pattern of infection. Mycopathologia. 1997;137:1–8.
4. Raghavendra KR et al. The nondermatophyte molds: emerging as leading cause of onychomycosis in south-east rajasthan. Indian Dermatol Online J. 2015;6(2):92–7. *PMC*. Web. 7 June 2016
5. Tosti A, Piraccini BM, Lorenzi S. Onychomycosis caused by non dermatophyte molds: clinical features and response to treatment of 7, cases. J Am Acad Dermatol. 2000;42(2pt1):217–24.
6. Morales-Cardona CA, Valbuena-Mesa MC, Alvarado Z, Solorzano-Amador A. Non-dermatophyte mould onychomycosis: a clinical and epidemiological study at a dermatology referral centre in Bogota, Colombia. Mycoses. 2013;57:284–93.
7. Finch J, Arenas R, Baran R. Fungal melanonychia. J Am Acad Dermatol. 2012;66:830–41.

8. Romano C, Paccagnini E, Difonzo EM. Onychomycosis caused by *Alternaria* spp. in Tuscany, Italy from 1985 to 1999. Mycoses. 2001;44:73–6.
9. Stephen S, Tosti A, Rubin AI. Diagnostic applications of nail clippings. Dermatol Clin. 2015;33(2):289–301.
10. Singal A, Khanna D. Onychomycosis: diagnosis and management. Indian J Dermatol Venereol Leprol. 2011;77:659–72.
11. Gupta AK, Drummond-Main C, Cooper EA, Brintnell W, Piraccini BM, Tosti A. Systematic review of nondermatophyte mold onychomycosis: diagnosis, clinical types, epidemiology, and treatment. J Am AcadDermatol. 2012;66(3):494–502.
12. Watanabe D, Kawamura C, Masuda Y, Akita Y, Tamada Y, Matsumoto Y, et al. successful treatment of toenail onychomycosis with photodynamic therapy. Arch Dermatol. 2008;144:19–21.
13. Donnelly RF, McCarron PA, Lightowler JM. Woolfson AD Bioadhesive patch-based delivery of 5-aminolevulinic acid to the nail for photodynamic therapy of onychomycosis. J Control Release. 2005;103(2):381–92.
14. Moreno G, Arenas R. Other fungi causing onychomycosis. Clin Dermatol. 2010;28:160–3.
15. Aspiroz C, ForuñoCebamanos B, Rezusta A, Paz-Crisóbal P, Domínguez-Luzón F, GenéDíaz J, Gilaberte Y. Photodynamic therapy for onychomycosis. Case report and review of the literature. Rev Iberoam Micol. 2011;28(4):191–3. Epub 2011 Apr 5
16. Gold MH. ALA-PDT and MAL-PDT: what makes them different. J Clin Aesthetic Derm. 2009;2(2):44–7.
17. Ranawaka RR, Nelun DS, Ragunathan RW. Non-dermatophyte mold onychomycosis in Sri Lanka. Dermatol Online J. 2012;18(1):7.
18. Nouripour-Sisakht S, Mirhendi H, Shidfar MR, et al. *Aspergillus* species as emerging causative agents of onychomycosis. J Mycol Med. 2015;25:101–7.
19. Greer DL. Evolving role of nondermatophytes in onychomycosis. Int J Dermatol. 1995;34:521–4.
20. Budak A, Macura AB, Mazur T, Laskownicka Z. Fungal species isolated from skin and nail lesions of the hands and feet of patients suspected of mycotic infection. Mykosen. 1987;30:434–9.
21. Arrese JE, Piérard-Franchimont C, Greimers R, Piérard GE. Fungi in onychomycosis. A study in immunohistochemistry and dual flow cytometry. J Eur Acad Dermatol Venereol. 1995;4:123–30.
22. Zaias N. Onychomycosis. Dermatol Clin. 1985;3:445–60.
23. Tosti A, Piraccini BM, Stinchi C, Lorenzi S. Onychomycosis due to Scopulariopsis brevicaulis: clinical features and response to systemic antifungals. Br J Dermatol. 1996;135:799–802.
24. Baran R, Tosti A, Piraccini BM. Uncommon clinical patterns of Fusarium nail infection: report of three cases. Br J Dermatol. 1997;136:424–7.
25. Tosti A, Piraccini BM. Proximal subungual onychomycosis due to Aspergillus niger. report of two cases. Br J Dermatol. 1998;139:156–7.
26. Piraccini BM, Tosti A. White superficial onychomycosis: epidemiological, clinical, and pathological study of 79 patients. Arch Dermatol. 2004;140:696–701.
27. Piraccini BM, Lorenzi S, Tosti A. 'Deep' white superficial onychomycosis due to mold. J Eur Acad Dermatol Venereol. 2002;16(5):532–3.
28. Baran R, Hay RJ, Tosti A, Haneke E. A new classification of onychomycosis. Br J Dermatol. 1998;139:567–71.
29. Rollman O, Johansson S. *Hendersonulatoruloidea* infection-successful response of onychomycosis to nail avulsion and topical ciclopiroxolamine. Acta Derm Venereol. 1987;67:506–10.
30. Ramani R, Ramani A, Kumari TGL, et al. Molds in onychomycosis. Int J Dermatol. 1993;32:877–8.
31. Escobar ML, Carmona-Fonseca J. Onychomycosis by common non-dermatophyte molds. Rev iberoamMicol. 2003;20:6–10.

32. Gupta AK, Jain HC, Lynde CW, Watteel GN, Summerbell RC. Prevalence and epidemiology of unsuspected onychomycosis in patients visiting dermatologists' offices in Ontario, Canada-a multicenter survey of 2001 patients. Int J Dermatol. 1997;36:783–7.
33. Godoy-Martinez P, Nunes FG, Tomimori-Yamashita J, Urrutia M, Zaror L, Silva V, et al. Onychomycosis in Sao Paulo Brazil. Mycopathologia. 2009;168:111–6.
34. Alvarez MI, Gonzalez LA, Castro LA. Onychomycosis in Cali Colombia. Mycopathologia. 2004;158:181–6.
35. Bokhari MA, Hussain I, Jahangir M, Haroon TS, Aman S, Khurshid K. Onychomycosis in Lahore Pakistan. Int J Dermatol. 1999;38:591–5.
36. Ungpakorn R, Lohaprathan S, Reangchainam S. Prevalence of foot diseases in outpatients attending the institute of Dermatology, Bangkok Thailand. Clin Exp Dermatol. 2004;29:87–90.
37. Gianni C, Cerri A, Crosti C. Non-dermatophytic onychomycosis: an underestimated entity? A study of 51 cases. Mycoses. 2000;43:29–33.
38. Ionnidou DJ, Maraki S, Krasagakis SK, Tosca A, Tselentis Y. The epidemiology of onychomycosis in Crete, Greece, between 1992 and 2001. J Eur Acad Dermatol Venereol. 2006;20:170–4.
39. Erbagci Z, Tuncel A, Zer Y, Balci I. A prospective epidemiological survery on the prevalence of onychomycosis and dermatophytosis in male boarding school residents. Mycopathologia. 2005;159:347–52.
40. Macura AB, Skóra M. 21-year retrospective study of the prevalence of *scopulariopsis brevicaulis* in patients suspected of superficial mycoses. Adv Dermatol Allergol. 2015;32(2):189–94.
41. Bassiri-Jahromi S, Khaksar AA. Nondermatophytic moulds as a causative agent of onychomycosis in Tehran. Indian J Dermatol. 2010;55:140–3.
42. Hilmioglu-Polat S, Metin DY, Inci R, Dereli T, Kilinc I, Tümbay E. Non-dermatophytic molds as agents of onychomycosis in Izmir, Turkey – A prospective study. Mycopathologia. 2005;160:125–8.
43. Bonifaz A, Cruz-Aguilar P, Ponce RM. Onychomycosis by molds. Report of 78 cases. Eur J Dermatol. 2007;17:70–2.
44. Farwa U, Abbasi SA, Mirza IA, et al. Non-dermatophyte moulds as pathogens of onychomycosis. J Coll Physicians Surg Pak. 2011;21:597–600.
45. Ghannoum MA, Hajjeh RA, Scher R. A large scale North American study of fungal isolates from nails: the frequency of onychomycosis, fungal distribution, and antifungal susceptibility patterns. J Am Acad Dermatol. 2000;43:641–8.

Chapter 8
Candida Onychomycosis

Edoardo Torres-Guerrero and Roberto Arenas

Key Features

- *Candida* species have emerged as second-line pathogens related to onychomycosis.
- *Candida* onychomycosis is increasingly found in individuals with defective immunity and that can be related with occupational aspects.
- *Candida* species is considered as one of the most important causes of fingernail onychomycosis, especially in women.
- The organism invades the nail plate and may cause paronychia, onycholysis, and melanonychia.
- The diagnostic route includes a complete interrogatory based on the patients' history: a physical examination and microscopy and culture of nail specimens.

Introduction

Onychomycosis is a fungal infection of nails that represents about 30 % of superficial mycotic infections. It is caused by dermatophytes, or non-dermatophytic molds, while *Candida* species have emerged as second-line pathogens [1]. This term is derived from the Greek words *onychos* (meaning nail) and *mycosis* (meaning fungal infection) [2]. But, it is traditionally referred to as non-dermatophytic infection of the nail, while *tinea unguium* specifically describes a dermatophytic invasion of the nail plate, but is now used as a general term to denote any fungal nail infection [3].

The importance of onychomycosis is often underestimated. In fact, onychomycosis can have significant negative effects on patients' emotional, social, and

E. Torres-Guerrero • R. Arenas (✉)
Mycology Section, Dr. Manuel Gea González General Hospital,
México, DF, México
e-mail: rarenas98@hotmail.com

A. Tosti et al. (eds.), *Onychomycosis*, DOI 10.1007/978-3-319-44853-4_8

occupational functioning and can, in addition, consume a sizable proportion of healthcare dollars. Affected patients may experience embarrassment in social and work situations, where they feel blighted or unclean, unwilling to allow their hands or feet to be seen [3]. Far more than being a simple cosmetic problem, infected nails serve as a chronic reservoir of infection which can give rise to repeated mycotic infections of the skin [4]. In spite of improved personal hygiene and living environment, onychomycosis continues to spread and persist [5].

Epidemiology

Onychomycosis encloses all fungal infections of the nail due to filamentous and yeast fungi, accounting for up to 50 % of all nail disorders which range from distal and lateral subungual, superficial, proximal subungual, and dystrophic onychomycosis; however, immunocompromised hosts can present a more significant health problem [6].

Over time, as the etiology of onychomycosis, yeasts from the genus *Candida* have emerged as important etiologic agents [7], so *Candida* onychomycosis is increasingly found in individuals having defective immunity consequential to aging, diabetes mellitus, vascular diseases, HIV infection, and drug therapies such as immunosuppressives and broad-spectrum antibiotics. Breached local immunity at the nail complex due to trauma, chronic exposure to moisture, and chemicals including smoke, detergents, soap, etc., also contributes to *Candida* onychomycosis [1]. Moreover, numerous factors exist for increasing the prevalence of onychomycosis in modern life such as wearing of shoes especially high-heeled shoes, high-moisture areas (gymnasium and wrestling mattresses by great numbers of people), use of broad-spectrum antibiotics, and corticosteroid therapy. *Candida* species is considered as one of the most important causes of fingernail onychomycosis, especially in women [6].

Candida onychomycosis constitutes an important health problem that can be related with occupational aspects, and this genus of yeasts may be the principal causative agent of fungal nail infections in some regions. Many authors around the world have documented that this condition affects mainly adult patients of female gender and toenails are more frequently involved than fingernails. The causative species varies around the world, and in some regions, non-*albicans* species have shown an increase of its frequency.

In a multicenter study conducted by Álvarez and colleagues in Colombia, from a total of 299 patients with nail lesions, onychomycosis was found in 183 cases (141 in toenails and 38 in fingernails), with a predominance in females (53 in males and 126 in females), and 4 cases in toenails and fingernails simultaneously (all females). Yeasts were identified in 40.7 % and *Candida albicans* was the most commonly isolated yeast species [8].

In a retrospective, observational, and descriptive study of fungal cultures conducted by Fich in Chile, specimens obtained from patients between December 2007 and December 2010 were analyzed. 29.1 % of cases with positive cultures were men and 70.9 % were women. *Candida* was retrieved from 467 of 8443 specimens (52 % fingernails and 48 % toenails), with a prevalence of 43.3 % for *C. parapsilosis*, while isolates of *Candida guilliermondii* were seen in 24.2 %, those of *Candida albicans* were present in 23.6 % of cases, those of *Candida* spp. were 4.3 %, and there were 4.71 % of cases of other isolates [9]. According to these data, Torres and colleagues in a retrospective study conducted in Mexico reported a frequency of *Candida* onychomycosis in 57.54 % of *Candida* mucocutaneous infections in a period of 6 years, with predominance in female gender of 65.49 % and a predilection of toenails' involvement in comparison with fingernails (86.01 % vs 13.99 %), and they reported a frequency of *C. albicans* in 42.80 %, *Candida krusei* in 28.41 %, *Candida tropicalis* in 15.86 %, and *Candida glabrata* in 12.91 % [10].

In a study with 140 patients conducted in Tehran, results show that females are more infected than males. The most common age group infected was 41–60 years (40.7 %). Toenails were affected more frequently than fingernails, and dystrophic onychomycosis was the most common clinical type (seen in 39.2 % of patients). Yeasts were the most frequent etiologic agents isolated (71.4 %), followed by non-dermatophytic molds in 17.1 % and dermatophytes in 11.5 % of patients [11]. According to these demographic data, in a study conducted in Paraiba, Brazil, from 1999 to 2010, women were the most affected by onychomycosis, which occur preferentially in adults, toenails are the favorite yeast targets, and the prevalent yeasts were *Candida tropicalis* and *C. krusei* [7].

Jesudanam et al., in India, studied 448 patients with nail abnormalities; and they reported *Candida* onychomycosis in 58.82 % of a total of 204 cases with positive direct microscopy, culture, or both, with a major prevalence in housewives (33.33 % of the total) [4]. Meanwhile, in Lebanon, Ellabib conducted a study with 500 patients. Yeasts of the genus *Candida* (*C. albicans*, *C. parapsilosis*, *C. glabrata*, *C. guilliermondii*, and *C. tropicalis*) were identified as the dominant agents in women (96 %); in contrast, dermatophytes were predominant in men (80 %) [12].

During a period of 10 years (2003–2012), Afshar et al. conducted a study in Iran with 1100 patients suspected with onychomycosis, and from 464 cultures, *Candida* spp. was isolated in 61.9 % of the cases, as the most common agents of onychomycosis [13].

On the other hand, Segal and colleagues analyzed epidemiologic parameters of onychomycosis in Israel. Data of a cohort of 27,093 patients, which were collected from six centers during a 10-year period, revealed that dermatophytes were the main causative agents of toenail onychomycosis, while *Candida parapsilosis* was the most frequent agent in women fingernails; and its frequency is increased with age [14]. A similar frequency of genera of causative agents was obtained by Seck et al. in Senegal, where dermatophytes predominate, but *Candida albicans* occupied the second position, with 90.86 % of isolated yeasts, and molds were isolated in nine cases (3.02 %) (all cases predominated in toenails) [15]. On the other hand, in a study conducted in Taiwan with 375 patients with onychomycosis, Chi et al. reported the isolation of dermatophytes in 227 patients (60.5 %), *Candida* in 118 (31.5 %), and molds in 30 (8 %) [16].

In Argentina, Nazar and colleagues studied 414 patients with onychopathies, and they reported a prevalence of the toenail and fingernail mycoses of 78 % and 58 %, respectively. The major etiologic agents were *Trichophyton rubrum*, *Candida* spp., and *Trichophyton mentagrophytes* [17].

Diabetic patients have a special predisposition to be affected with fungal infections and *Candida* onychomycosis as Imbert reports in Mexico. In an observational, descriptive, and transversal study made with 261 diabetic patients from public institutions of health of the state of Hidalgo, Mexico, he revealed onychomycosis was caused by *Candida guilliermondii*, *C. parapsilosis*, *C. glabrata*, *Candida* spp., and unidentified molds and yeasts [18].

Papini, in Italy, reported that diabetic patients showed onychomycosis in 53.3 % and foot skin mycosis in 46.7 % of the cases, with a prevalence of both fungal infections significantly higher than that observed in nondiabetic individuals. *Candida* spp., *Fusarium* spp., *Aspergillus* spp., and other molds were found in about 1/3 onychomycosis [19].

With respect to onychomycosis in childhood, in a study conducted in Korea with 59 children, 2.3 % of onychomycosis in general population is seen in children. In toenails, *Trichophyton rubrum* was reported in 51.3 %, followed by *Candida albicans* (10.2 %), *C. parapsilosis* (5.1 %), *C. tropicalis* (2.6 %), and *C. guilliermondii* (2.6 %); but in fingernails, *C. albicans* was the most common isolated pathogen (50.0 %) followed by *T. rubrum* (10.0 %) [20]. In another study, conducted by Gulgum in Turkey with 8122 schoolchildren (aged 5–16 years), culture-positive onychomycosis was detected in 27 cases, and yeasts were isolated in 10/27 cases (37.1 %), with a predominance of *Candida glabrata* (14.8 %) [21].

In a retrospective study conducted in Serbia, in a period from 2011 to 2015, out of 761 patients who underwent clinical and mycological examinations, 137 had *Candida* species isolated from nails. The dominant species was *Candida albicans* (36.59 %), *C. parapsilosis* (23.78 %), *C. krusei* (9.76 %), and *C. guilliermondii* (6.71 %) [22].

Clinical Features

The organism invades the entire nail plate and may cause other clinical syndromes, including onycholysis and paronychia. These forms occur more commonly in women and often affect the middle finger. It may be related with professional aspects where the repeated contact with water or humidity predisposes to this condition [3, 23]. *Candida* onychomycosis can be divided into three general categories:

1. Infection beginning as an infection of the structures surrounding the nail (paronychia). This is the most common type of *Candida* onychomycosis (Fig. 8.1). It starts as an edematous, reddened pad surrounding the nail plate; later, it can develop a periungual abscess. *Candida* spp. only penetrate the nail plate only secondarily after it has attacked the soft tissue around the nail

Fig. 8.1 Paronychia

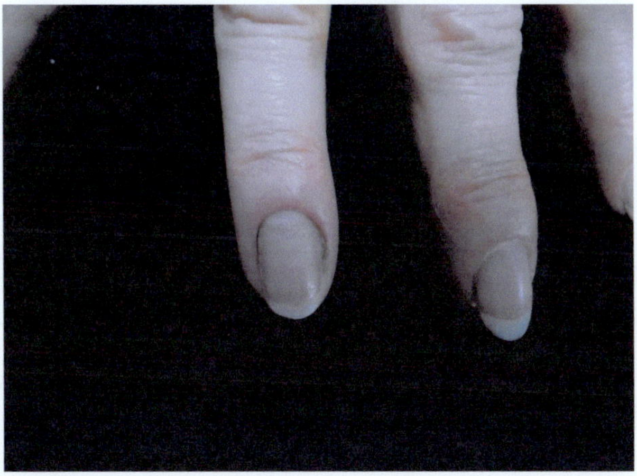

(unlike dermatophytic invasion). After infection of the nail matrix occurs, transverse depressions (Beau's lines) may appear in the nail plate, which becomes convex, rough, and, ultimately, dystrophic [3, 23].

2. *Candida* granuloma, which is more frequent in individuals with chronic mucocutaneous *Candida* infections, accounts for less than 1 % of onychomycosis cases. This condition is seen in immunocompromised patients and involves direct invasion of the nail plate, resulting, in advanced cases, in swelling of the proximal and lateral nail folds until the digit develops a pseudo-clubbing appearance.
3. Finally, *Candida* onycholysis. This form is more frequent in fingernails than toenails, and it occurs when the nail plate has separated from the nail bed. Distal subungual hyperkeratosis can be seen as a yellowish-gray mass that lifts off the nail plate. The lesion resembles that seen in patients with distal subungual onychomycosis [3].

Other clinical findings comprise fungal melanonychia (Fig. 8.2), with a greenish, brownish, or even black nail discoloration [23].

Diagnostic Clues

The diagnostic route of onychomycosis (caused by dermatophytes, *Candida* species, or other molds or yeasts) includes a complete interrogatory based on the patients' history: a physical examination and microscopy and culture of nail specimens [5].

The clinical presentation of dystrophic nails (with or without discoloration of the nail plate) should alert the clinician to the possibility of onychomycosis; however, it's necessary to use appropriate diagnostic techniques including direct microscopy and fungal culture to ensure correct diagnosis and treatment. The clinical appearance

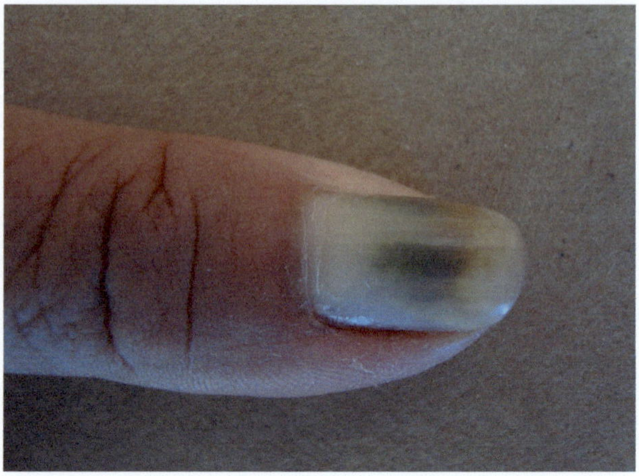

Fig. 8.2 Fungal melanonychia due to *Candida*

of the nail will help to recognize fungal from nonfungal etiologies of nail dystrophies. A detailed interrogation of patient's history can help to obtain information about predisposing factors for onychomycosis such as diabetes mellitus, older age, hyperhidrosis, professional occupations, hobbies, onychogryphosis, nail trauma, poor peripheral circulation, and immunosuppression [3].

Direct examination of a nail sample with potassium/sodium hydroxide (KOH or NaOH) or Chlorazol Black is the first step to support a clinical diagnosis of onychomycosis. The specimen is obtained by scraping of nail plate in its ventral portion (hyponychium), and it should be divided into two portions for direct microscopy and culture. To identify the causative agent, the laboratory culture of sampled material is necessary to identify the specific etiologic agent.

The specimen can be mounted in a solution of 20–25 % KOH or NaOH mixed with dimethyl sulfoxide and examined, first under ×10 and after under ×40 magnification (if a suggestive structure is present) (Fig. 8.3). When the sample is counterstained with chitin-specific Chlorazol Black, fungal structures are accentuated (it takes a dark green or blackish color); this is of particular value if the number of fungal elements is sparse, and it can help to discriminate contaminants such as cotton or elastic fibers, reducing the number of false-positive identifications [3, 23].

It is important to understand the limitations of direct microscopy in diagnosing the cause of onychomycosis, because this technique only serves as a screening test for the presence or absence of fungi, but it could be negative in approximately 15 % of cases, and this technique cannot identify the specific causative agents [3, 23]. Moreover, the sensitivity and specificity of this test are strongly influenced by the clinician's training. When examining a KOH preparation, the presence of round or ovoid spores suggests yeasts, but pseudohyphae or true hyphae could be present too. Almost half of all specimens taken from onychomycotic nails fail to yield a pathogen in culture. Other diagnostic techniques for a direct examination include Gram, Papanicolaou, Wright, or PAS (periodic acid-Schiff) stains or, in case of its availability, fluorescence microscopy with calcofluor white stain.

Fig. 8.3 Budding yeasts in direct microscopy (Chlorazol Black, 40X)

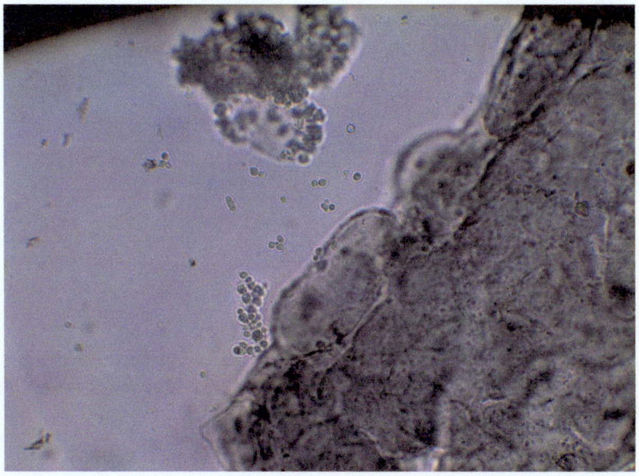

In onychomycosis, direct microscopy is the most efficient screening technique; however, careful matching of microscopic and culture results is necessary for the clinician to be confident of the diagnosis to avoid fungal resistance and therapeutic fails [3, 23].

Culture at room temperature (or at 37 ° C) is the only method by which the causative agents can be recognized. Routine culture media such as Sabouraud (with or without chloramphenicol), malt extract, or mycobiotic agar are adequate to obtain the fungal isolates, but cycloheximide inhibits the growth of *Candida parapsilosis*, *C. tropicalis*, *C. krusei*, and *C. zeylanoides*. The inoculation must be done rapidly because fungal and bacterial contaminants may obscure the real nail pathogen. After 28–72 h at 37 ° C, colonies grow. These organisms produce white, smooth, and brilliant colonies with a creamy consistence. The identification of *Candida* species is very important to establish the therapeutic regimen. Some chromogenic culture media have been developed to identify the most frequent *Candida* species. These include CHROMagar®, Biggy® (Fig. 8.4), or Candida-ID® media, and they can identify some species such as *Candida albicans*, *C. tropicalis*, *C. glabrata*, and *C. krusei* [23].

Other no routine laboratory tests to identify different *Candida* species include serum-induced filamentation (to recognize *C. albicans*), tetrazolium salt assays, and sensitivity to cycloheximide test.

Also, some systematic biochemical tests are available to identify some species, such as API 20C, API 32C, Vitek®, Uni-Yeast Tek®, Minitek®, Yeast-Ident®, and MicroScan®, which are based on the metabolic and physiologic characteristics of this genus of yeasts [23]. Other identification tools such as ViteK MS®, MALDI TOF/TOF®, and mass spectrometers are used to a wide range of fungi including *Candia* spp.

Nowadays, molecular diagnostics are a useful tool to specific identification of particular *Candida* species, and it can be helpful at the moment of deciding the antifungal regime, because some species have an intrinsic drug resistance.

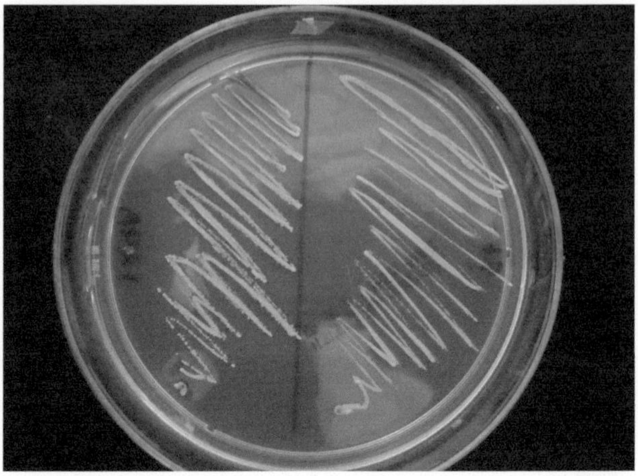

Fig. 8.4 Greenish colony of *Candida albicans* (CHROMagar® culture medium)

DNA sequencing-based tests are very specific to identify and differentiate among several species of *Candida* and other microorganisms. In some research centers of China, PCR-based assays combined with internal transcribed spacers sequencing such as ITS1-5.8S-ITS2 rDNA regions are performed to reveal the prevalence of *Candida* species including emerging species in onychomycosis [24, 25]. Other assay procedures consisted of PCR amplification of the ITS using universal primers, followed by hybridization of the digoxigenin-labeled amplicons to probes on the array [26]. For example, differentiation of *C. parapsilosis* complex species (*Candida parapsilosis* sensu stricto, *C. metapsilosis*, and *C. orthopsilosis*) is necessary, because *C. parapsilosis* has shown an intrinsic resistance to fluconazole in vitro. One method to help is the amplification of the secondary alcohol dehydrogenase (SADH) gene and digestion by the restriction enzyme Ban I [27].

However, the majority of these laboratory tools have a restricted availability, so a good clinical examination with a correct sampling of nail plate for direct microscopy and culture is still the most useful diagnostic strategy.

Summary for The Clinician

Onychomycosis encloses all fungal infections of the nail due to filamentous and yeast fungi, accounted for up to 50 % of all nail disorders. It is caused by dermatophytes or non-dermatophytic molds; however, *Candida* species have emerged as second-line pathogens, because *Candida* onychomycosis is increasingly found in individuals having defective immunity consequential to aging, diabetes mellitus, vascular diseases, HIV infection, and drug therapies such as immunosuppressives and broad-spectrum antibiotics. Moreover, numerous factors exist for increasing the prevalence of onychomycosis in modern life such as wearing of shoes especially high-heeled shoes, high-moisture areas (gymnasium and wrestling mattresses by great numbers of people), use of broad-spectrum antibiotics, and corticosteroid therapy. *Candida* onychomycosis constitutes an important health problem that also can be related with occupational aspects, and this genus of yeasts may be the principal causative agent of fungal nail infections in some regions. The causative species varies around the world, and in some regions, non-*albicans* species have showed an increase of its frequency.

The importance of onychomycosis is often underestimated. In fact, onychomycosis can have significant negative effects on patients' emotional, social, and occupational functioning and can, in addition, consume a sizable proportion of healthcare dollars. Far more than being a simple cosmetic problem, infected nails serve as a chronic reservoir of infection which can give rise to repeated mycotic infections of the skin. In spite of improved personal hygiene and living environment, onychomycosis continues to spread and persist.

Clinical Pearls

It may be related with immunosuppression or professional aspects where the repeated contact with water or humidity predisposes to this condition.

The organism causes three clinical syndromes: melanonychia, paronychia, and onycholysis.

Paronychia is the most common type of *Candida* onychomycosis.

Melanonychia adopts a greenish, brownish, or even black discoloration.

Candida granuloma is more frequent in individuals with chronic mucocutaneous *Candida* infections, and it appears as swelling of the proximal and lateral nail folds until the digit develops a pseudo-clubbing appearance.

The clinical presentation of dystrophic nails (with or without discoloration of the nail plate) should alert the clinician to the possibility of onychomycosis; however, it's necessary to use direct microscopy and fungal culture to ensure correct diagnosis and treatment.

References

1. Jayatilake JA, Tilakaratne WM, Panagoda GJ. Candida onychomycosis: a mini-review. Mycopathologia. 2009;168(4):165–73.
2. Martínez-Herrera EO, Arroyo-Camarena S, Tejada-García DL, Porras-López CF, Arenas R. Onychomycosis due to opportunistic molds. An Bras Dermatol. 2015;90(3):334–7.
3. Elewski BE. Onychomycosis: pathogenesis, diagnosis, and management. Clin Microbiol Rev. 1998;11(3):415–29.

4. Jesudanam TM, Rao GR, Lakshmi DJ, Kumari GR. Onychomycosis: a significant medical problem. Indian J Dermatol Venereol Leprol. 2002;68(6):326–9.
5. Kaur R, Kashyap B, Bhalla P. Onychomycosis–epidemiology, diagnosis and management. Indian J Med Microbiol. 2008;26(2):108–16.
6. Mohammadi R, Badiee P, Badali H, Abastabar M, Safa AH, Hadipour M, Yazdani H, Heshmat F. Use of restriction fragment length polymorphism to identify *Candida* species, related to onychomycosis. Adv Biomed Res. 2015;4:95.
7. Arrua JM, Rodrigues LA, Pereira FO, Lima EO. Prevalence of *Candida tropicalis* and *Candida krusei* in onychomycosis in João Pessoa, Paraiba, Brazil from 1999 to 2010. An Acad Bras Cienc. 2015;87(3):1819–22.
8. Alvarez MI, González LA, Castro LA. Onychomycosis in Cali, Colombia. Mycopathologia. 2004;158(2):181–6.
9. Fich F, Abarzúa-Araya A, Pérez M, Nauhm Y, León E. *Candida parapsilosis* and *Candida guillermondii*: *emerging pathogens in nail candidiasis*. Indian J Dermatol. 2014;59(1):24–9.
10. Torres – Guerrero E, del Vasquez ME, Arenas R. Infecciones por *Candida* spp. Datos clínico-epidemiológicos y de tipificación de *Candida* en un hospital de segundo nivel. Dermatología CMQ. 2014;12(1):18–23.
11. Soltani M, Khosravi AR, Shokri H, Sharifzadeh A, Balal A. A study of onychomycosis in patients attending a dermatology center in Tehran,Iran. J Mycol Med. 2015;25(2):e81–7.
12. Ellabib MS, Agaj M, Khalifa Z, Kavanagh K. Yeasts of the genus *Candida* are the dominant cause of onychomycosis in Libyan women but not men: results of a 2-year surveillance study. Br J Dermatol. 2002;146(6):1038–41.
13. Afshar P, Khodavaisy S, Kalhori S, Ghasemi M, Razavyoon T. Onychomycosis in north-East of iran. Iran J Microbiol. 2014;6(2):98–103.
14. Segal R, Shemer A, Hochberg M, Keness Y, Shvarzman R, Mandelblat M, Frenkel M, Segal E. Onychomycosis in Israel: epidemiological aspects. Mycoses. 2015;58(3):133–9.
15. Seck MC, Ndiaye D, Diongue K, Ndiaye M, Badiane AS, Sow D, Sylla K, Tine R, Ndiaye JL, Faye B, Ndir O. Mycological profile of onychomycosis in Dakar (Senegal). J Mycol Med. 2014;24(2):124–8.
16. Chi CC, Wang SH, Chou MC. The causative pathogens of onychomycosis in southern Taiwan. Mycoses. 2005;48(6):413–20.
17. Nazar JR, Gerosa PE, Díaz OA. Onychomycoses: epidemiology, causative agents and assessment of diagnostic laboratory methods. Rev Argent Microbiol. 2012;44(1):21–5.
18. Imbert JL, G Gomez JV, Escudero RB, Blasco JL. Onychomycosis by yeast not common in diabetics of a health center. Semergen. 2015;42(7):449–57 pii: S1138-3593(15)00307-X. doi: 10.1016/j.semerg.2015.08.006. [Epub ahead of print].
19. Papini M, Cicoletti M, Fabrizi V, Landucci P. Skin and nail mycoses in patients with diabetic foot. G Ital Dermatol Venereol. 2013;148(6):603–8.
20. Kim DM, Suh MK, Ha GY. Onychomycosis in children: an experience of 59 cases. Ann Dermatol. 2013;25(3):327–34.
21. Gulgun M, Balci E, Karaoglu A, Kesik V, Babacan O, Fidanci MK, Turker T, Tok D, Koc N. Prevalence and risk factors of onychomycosis in primary school children living in rural and urban areas in Central Anatolia of Turkey. Indian J Dermatol Venereol Leprol. 2013;79(6):777–82.
22. Otašević S, Barac A, Pekmezovic M, Tasic S, Ignjatović A, Momčilović S, Stojanović P, Arsic Arsenijevic V, Hay R. The prevalence of *Candida* onychomycosis in Southeastern Serbia from 2011 to 2015. Mycoses. 2016;59(3):167–72.
23. Arenas R. Micología médica Ilustrada. 5th ed. México: McGraw Hill Companies; 2014. p. 239–60.
24. Feng X, Ling B, Yang X, Liao W, Pan W, Yao Z. Molecular Identification of *Candida* Species isolated from onychomycosis in Shanghai,China. Mycopathologia. 2015;180(5-6):365–71.

25. Galán-Sánchez F, García-Agudo L, García-Martos P, Rodríguez-Iglesias M. *Candida galli* as a cause of tinea unguium-molecular characterization of a rare clinical fungal entity. Mycopathologia. 2014;178(3-4):303–6.
26. Han HW, Hsu MM, Choi JS, Hsu CK, Hsieh HY, Li HC, Chang HC, Chang TC. Rapid detection of dermatophytes and *Candida albicans* in onychomycosis specimens by an oligonucleotide array. BMC Infect Dis. 2014;14:581.
27. Ataides FS, Costa CR, Souza LK, Fernandes O, Jesuino RS, Silva Mdo R. Molecular identification and antifungal susceptibility profiles of *Candida parapsilosis* complex species isolated from culture collection of clinical samples. Rev Soc Bras Med Trop. 2015;48(4):454–9.

Chapter 9
Pigmented Onychomycosis (Fungal Melanonychia)

Pablo Campos-Macias and Roberto Arenas

Key Features
Fungal melanonychia is a variety of onychomycosis. It is caused by dematiaceous fungi and rarely by yeasts and non-dermatophyte molds. Its main feature is brown to black pigmentation of the nail.

A full medical history is required for diagnosis. Due to the great number of causative agents, a complete mycological examination is necessary (dermoscopy, KOH, culture, and, in some cases, histopathology, immunohistochemistry, and flow cytometry).

Fungal melanonychia is usually resistant to most antifungal agents.

Melanonychia is defined as a brown or black pigmentation of the nail unit and has different etiologies; when caused by fungi, it is termed fungal melanonychia (Fig. 9.1).

Fungal melanonychia is an infrequent complication of onychomycosis [1].

Onychomycosis is the invasion of nails by fungi, regardless of its individual causative agents. Fungal melanonychia is a clinical variety of onychomycosis. It is most often caused by opportunistic filamentous pigmented fungi (also known as phaeoid or dematiaceous) and sometimes by non-dematiaceous agents which include some dermatophytes (*Aspergillus* spp.) and *Candida* spp. [1–3].

P. Campos-Macias
Dermatology, Aranda de la Parra, Hidalgo 326, León, Guanajuato, Mexico

R. Arenas (✉)
Mycology Section, Dr. Manuel Gea González General Hospital,
México, DF, México
e-mail: rarenas98@hotmail.com

A. Tosti et al. (eds.), *Onychomycosis*, DOI 10.1007/978-3-319-44853-4_9

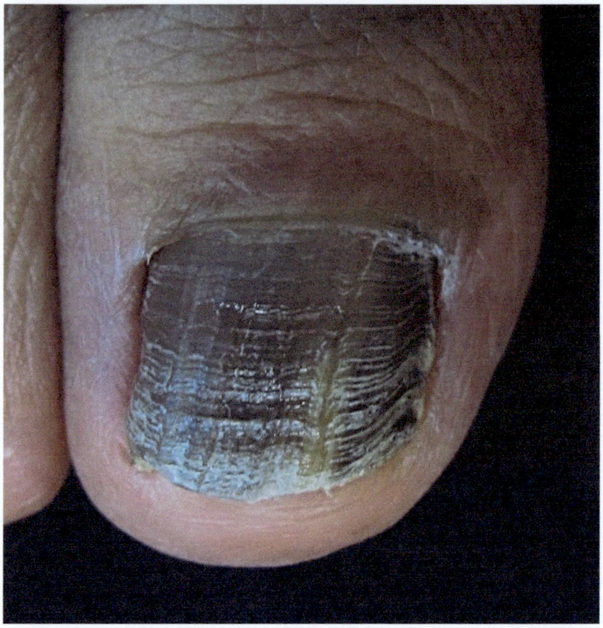

Fig. 9.1 Fungal melanonychia

Epidemiology

The fungal pathogens that cause fungal melanonychia are ubiquitous and become more common in areas close to the equator. Soil is their natural habitat, where they act as saprophytes or as plant pathogens, inhabiting decaying wood or polluted water. They are endemic in tropical and subtropical regions. In humans, their presence increases with age, as a consequence of slower nail growth, deteriorated immunity, sedentarism, and difficulty in observing proper foot care [4]. They are more frequent in men than women and in toenails. Subcutaneous and systemic phaeoid fungal infections occur in immunosuppressed hosts, but superficial and localized infections, such as nail infections, occur in immunocompetent hosts and are not usually contagious. Infections caused by dermatophytes and yeasts can occur both in immunosuppressed and immunocompetent hosts [1, 5].

Etiology and Pathogenesis

Unlike dermatophytes, non-dermatophyte molds (NDM) are not keratinolytic and affect nonkeratinized intercellular cement. They act as opportunistic pathogens, causing infection only when keratin has been disrupted by dermatophytes, trauma, or other nail diseases [6].

Table 9.1 Phaeoid agents of fungal melanonychia

Acrothecium nigrum	*Exophiala* species
Alternaria species	*Exophiala (Wangiella) jeanselmei*
Alternaria alternata	*Exophiala (Wangiella) dermatitidis*
Alternaria chlamydospora	*Exophiala Hongkongensis*
Alternaria tenuis	*Exophiala bergeri*
Alternaria humícola	*Exophiala oligosperma*
Alternaria pluriseptata	*Fusarium oxysporum*
Aureobasidium pullulans (possible case)	*Hormodendrum elatum*
Botryodiplodia (*Lasiodiplodia*) *theobromae*	*Microascus desmosporus*
Chaetomium perpulchrum	*Phyllostictina sydow*
Cladosporium (*Cladophialophora*) *carrionii*	*Pyrenochaeta unguis-hominis*
Cladosporium sphaerospermum	*Nattrassia mangiferae*
Curvularia lunata	*Scytalidium* species
	Scytalidium dimidiatum
	Scytalidium hyalinum
Non-phaeoid agents of fungal melanonychia	
Aspergillus niger	*Candida* species
Blastomyces	*Candida albicans*
Dermatophytes	*Candida humicola*
Trichophyton rubrum	*Candida parapsilosis*
Trichophyton soudanense	*Candida tropicalis*

Dermatophytes are keratinophilic fungi whose presence is limited to structures containing keratin. Local factors such as humid work environments or nail trauma, or systemic factors, may promote the growth of *Candida* and similar yeasts.

NDM cause 1.5–17.5 % of onychomycoses [7]. A 2012 report by Finch et al. lists 29 causative agents: 21 dematiaceous species and 8 non-dematiaceous species [1]. A year later, Patrick and Woo reported three new *Exophiala* species [8–9] (Table 9.1).

Neoscytalidium dimidiatum (*formerly Scytalidium dimidiatum*) is the most isolated dematiaceous fungus in cases of fungal melanonychia; a mutant nonpigmented variety, *S. hyalinum*, has also been described [10–12]. These are thermotolerant fungi found in nature as pathogens in trees, vineyards, and root vegetables. Their presence has been documented in several countries, and they are endemic in two zones: Southeast Asia, mainly in Thailand, and the Caribbean, especially in Trinidad and Tobago, with a prevalence of 41–45 %. In Europe and the USA, they have been found mostly in migrants from tropical areas. Some cases have been reported in India, Far East, France, the UK, Spain, and Africa. Most infections by dematiaceous fungi are limited to the nails and skin, with clinical features resembling those of dermatophyte infections. KOH shows filaments of varying thickness, with a double contour because of the retraction of the cytoplasm from the cell wall. Cycloheximide-containing media impair their growth. Colonies grow rapidly in culture, and dematiaceous varieties show a gray to black pigmentation. Microscopically, chains of arthroconidia often appear branched, with thick walls that are sometimes bicellular and a hue from hyaline to dark [2].

Alternaria alternata is the *Alternaria* species most frequently isolated in cases of ungual melanonychia. It is a common fungus in soil, manure, plants (*chrysanthemums*, strawberries, tomatoes, carrots, *asparagus*), wood, and foods. The presence of conidia in the air and in damp environments makes it a common allergen. *Alternaria* can cause superficial skin and nail lesions, but extracutaneous diseases are very rare. Direct KOH examination reveals slightly irregular pigmented filaments. Colonies in culture are dark colored, with a wooly or dusty appearance. Their microscopic features are long, straight, pigmented conidiophores with brown, smooth-walled, and septated muriform conidia with a round base and a sharp apex, isolated or in chains [13–15].

Less common dematiaceous fungi include some species of *Exophiala* found in carbohydrate-rich and humid environments (polluted water, restrooms, sauna). Prior to 2012, four cases of onychomycosis caused by *E. dermatitidis* and three cases caused by *E. jeanselmei* had been reported. In 2013, Patrick and Woo reported an additional four cases, including the first known case associated with *E. hongkongensis*, *E. bergeri*, and *E. oligosperma* [8].

Other dematiaceous fungi have been reported to cause melanonychia (Table 9.1).

Among the non-dematiaceous fungi, *Trichophyton rubrum* is the most frequently isolated agent of fungal melanonychia [1]. It has been reported that strains can produce a diffusible black pigment [16, 17].

Further studies have shown that dermatophytes, including *T. mentagrophytes*, *T. rubrum*, *E. floccosum*, and *M. gypseum*, can synthesize melanin or melanin-like pigments when grown in vitro and that these pigments are present in septate hyphae in dermatophyte-infected skin; however, there is no available data to suggest that melanin plays a critical role in the pathogenesis of dermatophytosis [18].

Aspergillus niger has been reported to cause diffuse, black melanonychia, and subungual onychomycosis [19–21].

Species of *Candida* isolated in cases of melanonychia include *Candida albicans*, *Candida humicola*, *Candida tropicalis*, and *Candida parapsilosis* [22–25]. In 2005 Morris-Jones demonstrated the synthesis of melanin by *Candida albicans* both in vitro and in active infection [26].

Biological Features of Pigmented Fungi

Seyedmojtaba Seyedmousavi's 2014 review of the biology of black yeasts and their filamentous relatives identifies virulence factors.

Melanins are high-molecular-weight brown to black pigments found in human beings, plants, and fungi alike, although with variable molecular structure and synthesis. The melanin pigment is believed to contribute to the organism's ability to elude host immune responses through blocking the effects of hydrolytic enzymes on the cell wall and scavenging free radicals liberated by phagocytic cells during the oxidative burst. The presence of melanin has an inhibitory effect on receptor-mediated phagocytosis, interfering with nitric oxide production, and protects black yeast from destruction by host cells in vitro. Also mechanism of carotenoid action is more likely to consist of shielding sensitive molecules or organelles than of neutralization of harmful oxidants.

Chitin syntheses are considered cell wall-associated virulence factors, because cell walls of fungi act as initial protective barrier against potential hostile environment. Chitin, an unbranched beta-1,4-linked homopolymer of *N*-acetylglucosamine (GlcNAc), is a structural component of the fungal cell wall and plays important roles in cellular development, structural morphogenesis, spore formation, and the maintenance of cell wall integrity.

The development of pigmented muriform cells is an important virulence factor for black yeasts and their filamentous relatives. The presence of this form of reproduction is thought to be an adaptation to harsh environmental conditions, such as low temperature, low water availability, acidity, nutrient deficiency, high UV exposure, high salt concentrations, or high temperature.

Black yeast species that are able to grow at temperatures of 37 °C or higher (thermotolerance) may cause systemic or disseminated infections in mammals, while those with maximum growth temperatures (35–37 °C) cause subcutaneous and superficial infections in humans.

Cell wall hydrophobicity and adhesion may be factors for pathogenesis of some black yeasts and their filamentous relatives. Inside the host, infectious propagules adhere to epithelial cells and differentiate into muriform cells, which effectively resist destruction by host effector cells and allow the establishment of chronic disease. This phenomenon may be enhanced by relative cellular hydrophobicity due to the presence of hydrophilic extracellular polysaccharides.

Host defense against black yeasts and their filamentous relatives has been shown to rely mainly on the ingestion and elimination of fungal cells by cells of the innate immune system, especially neutrophils and macrophages. A failure in innate recognition can result in chronic features that highlight the lack of pattern recognition receptor signaling. Cell-mediated immunity is more critical than a humoral immune response for host defense against diseases caused by black yeasts and their filamentous. Severe forms are characterized by elevated production of IL-4 and IL-10. These mediators, associated with low IFN-γ and lymphocyte proliferation levels, may result in a depressed cellular immune response. In contrast, patients with the mild form represent the opposite pole, in which high-level IFN-γ production parallels lymphocyte proliferation, in addition to very low levels of IL-10 [27].

Clinical Features

The clinical manifestation of fungal melanonychia is typically brown to black discoloration (Fig. 9.1). Also dystrophic nails, onycholysis, thickening, subungual hyperkeratosis and paronychia can be observed. The clinical pattern of nail involvement can raise clues as the origin of infection. Distal and lateral subungual onychomycosis

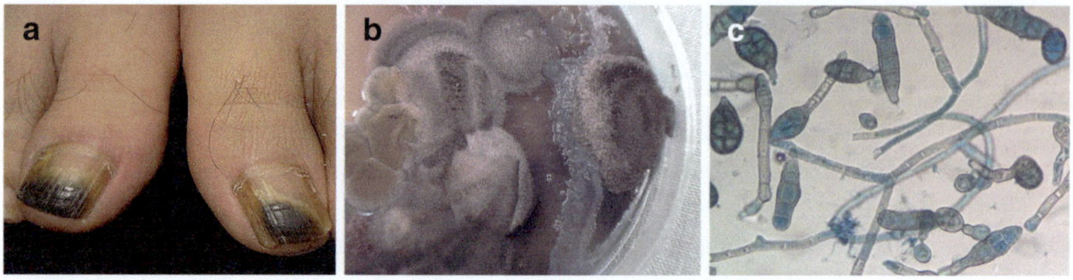

Fig. 9.2 (**a**) Melanonychia caused by *Alternaria alternata*, (**b**) dark-colored colonies with a cotton-like aspect, (**c**) pigmented conidiophores with muriform conidia

is the most common clinical pattern of nail infection. In *Neoscytalidium* species affection nails can become markedly thickened, and keratinous debris can be collects under the nail [1]. Distal subungual onychomycosis and occasionally distal onycholysis are the clinical patterns of nail infection by *Alternaria* [13, 28, 29] (Fig. 9.2a–c). Longitudinal or distal melanonychia is more common with strains of dermatophyte such as *T. rubrum* [1] (Fig. 9.3).

When fungal nail infection produces longitudinal melanonychia, the band of pigmentation is typically wider distally and tapers proximally, consistent with distal-to-proximal extension of infection.

Proximal subungual onychomycosis, with infection beginning at the proximal nail fold and extending distally, is a common presentation of onychomycosis as a result of non-dermatophyte molds. It is often associated with paronychia, and the more common pathogen microorganism is *Candida*; although this yeast is capable of melanin synthesis, nail pigmentation more commonly results from activation of host melanocytes caused by paronychial inflammation more common in darker skin phototypes [1, 7, 26, 30] (Fig. 9.4a–c). Proximal subungual onychomycosis with periungual inflammation by *Neoscytalidium* can be observed [11].

Black superficial onychomycosis is commonly caused by *Trichophyton rubrum* and *Neoscytalidium* spp. *Aspergillus* onychomycosis typically involves a superficial white pattern but can appear as proximal subungual onychomycosis, striated deep leukonychia or dark spots, and diffuse melanonychia. The black discoloration is likely from *A. niger's* darkly colored pigment aspergillin [21]. It is frequently accompanied by periungual inflammation and black pigmentation of the proximal nail fold [20, 31].

Any of the above clinical patterns of onychomycosis may lead to complete destruction of the nail, known as total nail dystrophy [1] (Fig. 9.5).

Diagnosis

Diagnoses of fungal melanonychia cannot be made on the basis of clinical observation alone. Direct microscopy examination (KOH or chlorazol black E® Delasco, Council Bluffs, IA) plays an important role in diagnosing nail fungal infections and confirms infection by ascertaining the presence of fungal hyphae/filaments or yeast

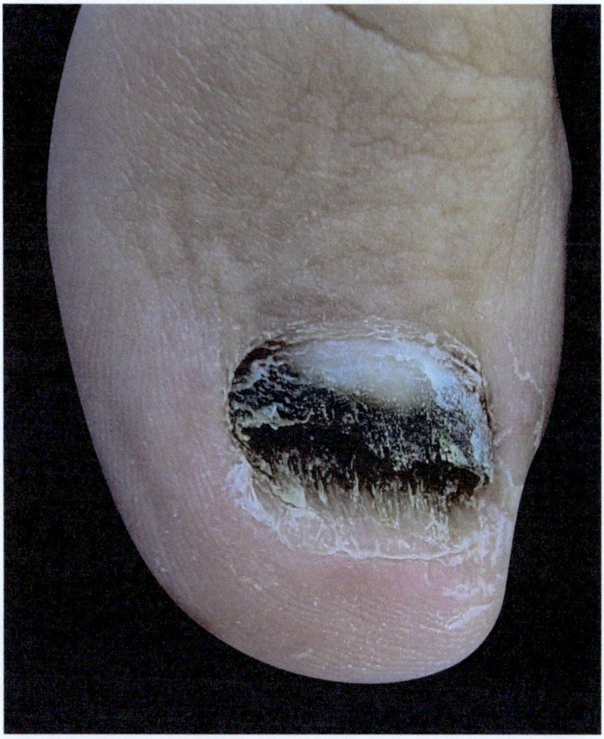

Fig. 9.3 Melanonychia caused by *Trichophyton rubrum*

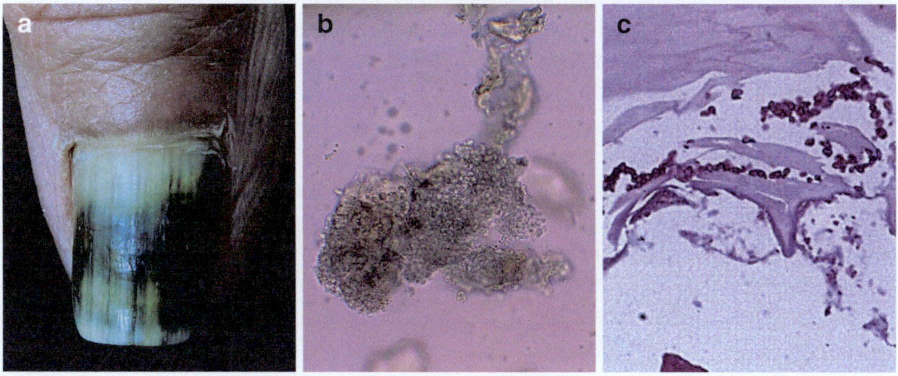

Fig. 9.4 (**a**) Melanonychia caused by *Candida parapsilosis*; (**b**) direct examination shows yeasts; (**c**) evidence of yeasts in histopathological examination

pseudohyphae (Fig. 9.4b); with dematiaceous organisms, the pigmentation is often clearly seen in direct microscopy. However, fungal cultures are the only definitive test that can be used to identify the genus and the species on the infectious organism (Fig. 9.2b). Fungal cultures are the most important method for identification of the causative organism. The use of cycloheximide-containing media must be avoided, as it inhibits the growth of dematiaceous and opportunistic fungi. Demonstrating

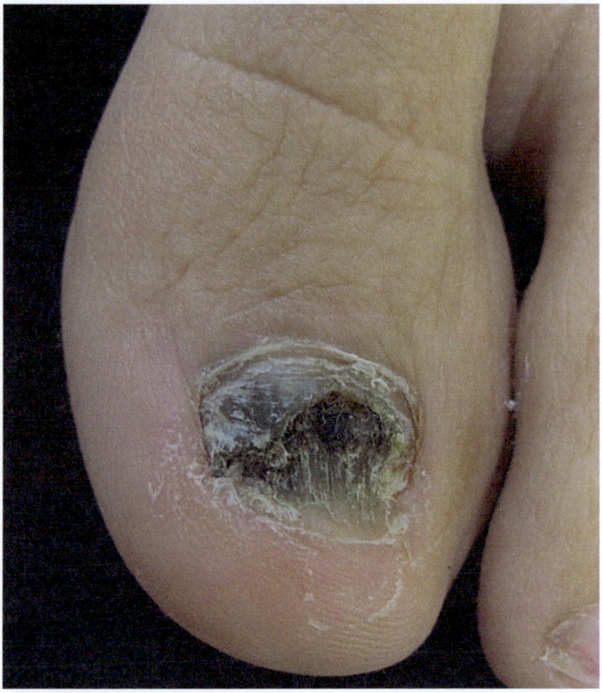

Fig. 9.5 Melanonychia caused by *Trichophyton rubrum*, total nail dystrophy

that a dematiaceous mold is the causative agent of melanonychia can be challenging because these species are common environmental contaminants or secondarily colonizing agents. Since molds are common contaminants in the laboratory, cultures from consecutively taken nail scrapings should be made and carefully evaluated in order to diagnose a mold onychomycosis. The criteria set forth by English can be helpful in establishing the pathogenicity of NDM in onychomycosis [1, 6].

Exceptionally histologic analysis of nail biopsy specimens is necessary for defining the nature and localization of fungi in the nail plate (Fig. 9.4c). Immunohistochemistry and flow cytometry can lead us prominent information about identification of fungi [32].

Dermoscopy is a noninvasive method that helps to narrow the differential diagnosis of ungual pigmented lesions and can assist in the recognition of fungal melanonychia [33].

Differential Diagnosis

The observation of a black-brown pigmentation of the nail is often alarming for the patient and for the clinician, as they are aware that it can be a possible clinical manifestation of melanoma of the nail apparatus. Nail melanoma is not the most common cause of nail melanonychia. However, the severity of this malignancy and the importance of early diagnosis in its treatment place it at the center of differential diagnosis.

Because a multiplicity of factors can cause nail pigmentation, a careful study protocol should be followed in these cases. For a detailed summary of the differential diagnosis of nail pigmentation, see the excellent article by Piraccini et al. [34].

Nail pigmentation may be secondary to endogenous or exogenous factors. A detailed patient history is a crucial part of the clinical examination. It is important to investigate occupational exposure, athletic activities, and past medical history, including systemic or cutaneous diseases, medication, the time and manner of pigmentation appearance, its evolution, and accompanying symptoms. Physical examination should be conducted in a well-lit area, all nails should be examined, and the number of affected nails should be recorded.

Nail evaluation must include the nail plate and the periungual tissues, including the distal pulp, and should be done moving the digit, so as to look at it frontally, laterally, and from below [34].

Nail pigment of non-melanocytic origin (nail hyperchromia).

Exogenous Pigmentation

Among the most frequent causes of exogenous pigmentation are contact with chemical agents, topical application of therapeutic agents such as silver nitrate, tobacco, and cosmetics [35].

Subungual hematoma usually appears as a reddish to reddish-black pigment depending on the age of the bleed. By dermoscopy we are able to identify small reddish to reddish-black globules along the proximal and lateral margins of the pigment. The distal part will often have streaks of pigment. The pigment is homogenous and no melanin granules can be observed. The hematoma will progressively grow out distally as the nail plate grows (Fig. 9.6a, b). Any subungual hemorrhage that does not grow out with the nail or that recurs at the same place requires special attention [34–36].

Nail Pigmentation of Melanocytic Origin

Longitudinal melanonychia (ML) is a result of focal melanocytic activation.

Racial longitudinal melanonychia is present in 80 % of Afro-Americans, 50 % of Hispanics, and 10–30 % of Japanese and is observed in dark-skinned individuals with skin types V and VI, especially those over 60 years of age; they can present as single or more often multiple bands involving one or more digits (Fig. 9.7).

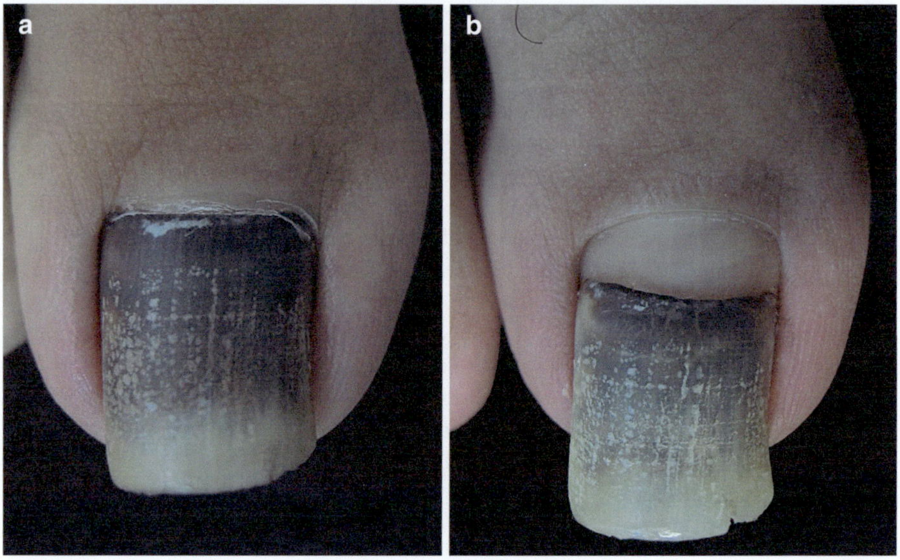

Fig. 9.6 (**a**) Subungual hematoma; (**b**) the hematoma will move distally as the nail plate grows

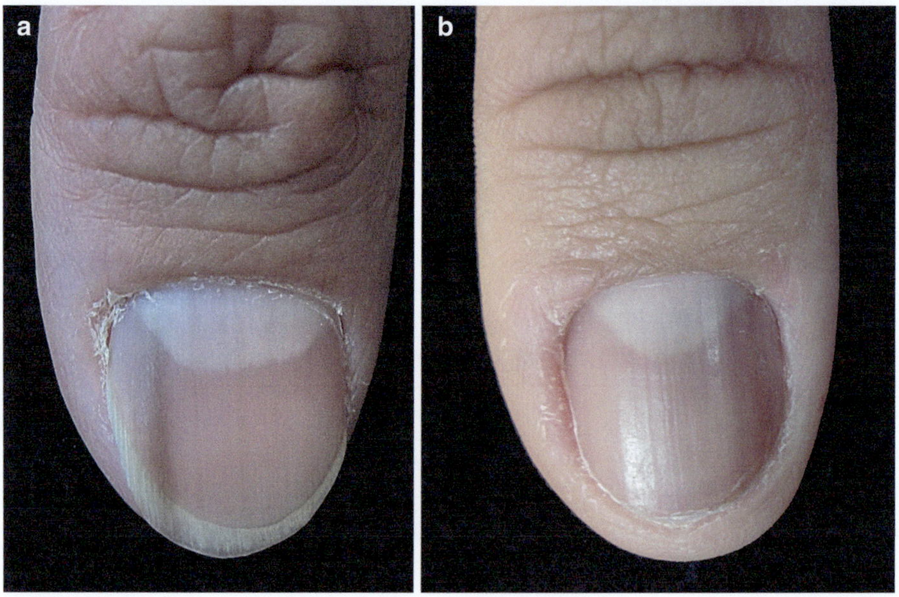

Fig. 9.7 (**a**) Racial longitudinal melanonychia; (**b**) melanonychia striata

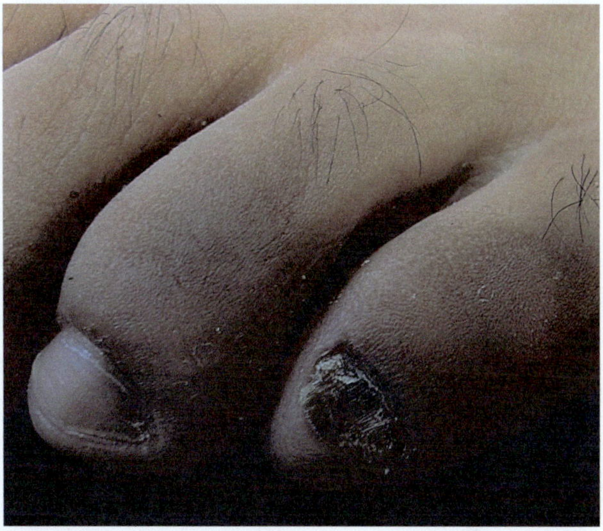

Fig. 9.8 Frictional melanonychia of the fifth toe

The more frequent manifestation of traumatic longitudinal melanonychia is melanonychia which involves the fourth and fifth toenails that undergo friction with the shoes, more frequent in women (Fig. 9.8). Melanonychia due to auto-induced nail diseases is associated with signs of mechanical damage of nail matrix, nail plate, or periungual tissues.

Drug longitudinal melanonychia is due to chemotherapeutic drugs, the most common of which are daunorubicin, methotrexate, etoposide, cytarabine, cyclophosphamide, and hydroxyurea [37–41] (Fig. 9.9).

Inherited diseases such as Laugier-Hunziker syndrome is an acquired disorder of the pigment system. The characteristic findings include longitudinal melanonychia and macular pigmentation of the lips, mouth, and anogenital area [42, 43].

Endocrine longitudinal melanonychia is nail pigmentation during pregnancy [44]. It occurs as a manifestation of Addison's disease or pituitary adenoma [45, 46].

Longitudinal melanonychia may be associated with inflammatory nail disorders such as psoriasis or lichen planus or autoimmune diseases like systemic lupus erythematosus and localized scleroderma [47–49].

Longitudinal melanonychia is a result of non-melanocytic nail tumors that activate melanocytes resulting in the formation of a longitudinal pigmented nail band, such as Bowen disease [50, 51], squamous cell carcinoma [52, 53], and subungual basal cell carcinoma [54].

Nail pigmentation is a result of melanocytic proliferation.

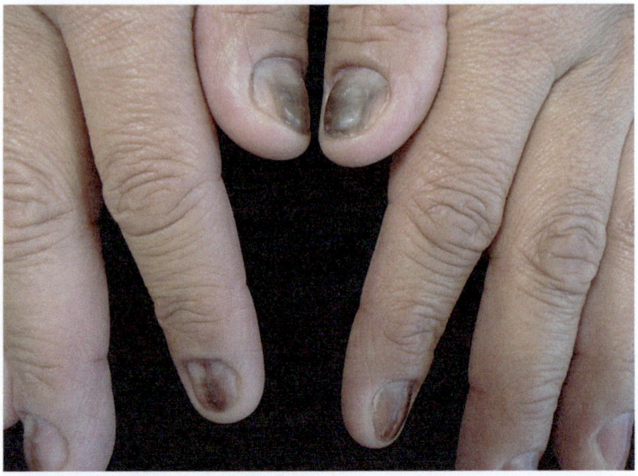

Fig. 9.9 Melanonychia due to chemotherapy

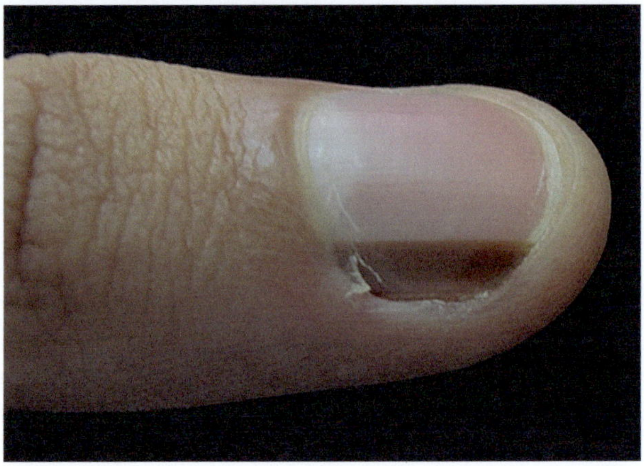

Fig. 9.10 Subungual nevus in a schoolchild

Longitudinal melanonychia of one nail is not associated with nail lesions that explain its appearance; onset in childhood is in most of the cases due to nail matrix nevus (Fig. 9.9). Nail melanoma is exceedingly rare in children [55–57].

Adult-onset melanonychia of a single digit is an alarming sign which should be carefully evaluated for melanoma (Fig. 9.10). As many as two thirds of ungual melanomas begin with brown to black pigmentation of the nail. In 2000, Eyal K Levit and his group established six criteria to improve early detection and thus survival of subungual melanoma, namely, ABCDEF of subungual melanoma [58], of which Piraccini emphasizes items A, B, and E. *A* stands for *a*ge (peak incidence being in the fifth to seventh decades of life and *A*frican-Americans, *A*sians, and native *A*mericans in whom subungual melanoma accounts for up to one third of all melanoma cases); *B* stands for brown to black band with breadth of 3 mm or more and variegated borders and *E* stands for *e*xtension of the pigment onto the proximal and/or lateral nail fold (i.e., Hutchinson's sign) (Fig. 9.11). Fungal melanonychia

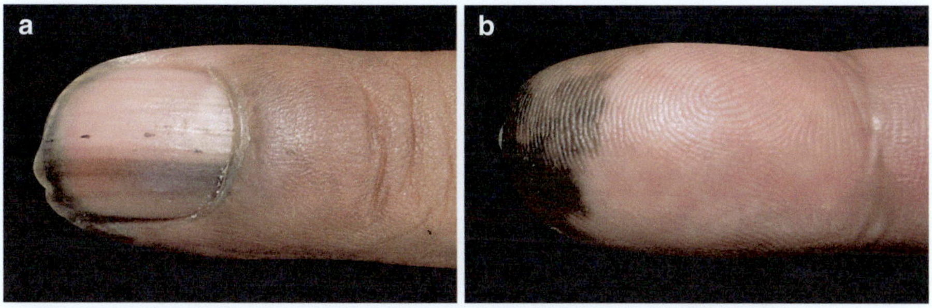

Fig. 9.11 Melanoma. (**a**) Adult-onset linear melanonychia; (**b**) Hutchinson's sign

may clinically mimic subungual melanoma, so an accurate, timely diagnosis is of first importance. Dermatoscopy can be a useful diagnostic tool when performed by experienced personnel; certain variables, such as nails that are extremely thick or completely black, can yield false results. The definitive diagnosis of subungual melanoma is made by biopsy.

Treatment

Black nail pigmentation is a distressing symptom, and many patients seek medical attention for fear that it may be a sign of malignancy. When cancer is ruled out and a diagnosis of fungal melanonychia is established, some patients choose not to pursue treatment (Fig. 9.12).

The treatment of onychomycosis due to non-dermatophytic molds is difficult, as there is today no consensus. The choice of an antifungal agent will first depend on the species that is involved in the infection but also on the severity of nail lesions and on the patient himself. In most cases the onychomycosis will be cured with chemical or mechanical removing of the infected tissues, followed by a local antifungal treatment. In some cases, a systemic therapy will be discussed [59].

Treatment of *Neoscytalidium dimidiatum* infection is exceptionally difficult, as it does not respond to griseofulvin, ketoconazole, fluconazole, itraconazole, or terbinafine [60]. A report by Tosti lists the outcomes of treatment in 431 cases of onychomycosis, including 59 cases caused by molds. A variety of treatments were used (systemic itraconazole, systemic terbinafine, topical terbinafine following nail plate avulsion, and ciclopirox nail lacquer), resulting in the cure of 69.2 % of *S. brevicaulis* cases, 71.4 % of *Acremonium* cases, and 40 % of *Fusarium* cases. The study concludes that topical therapy may prove more successful than systemic therapy in these cases. Regarding infection by *Aspergillus*, the study reports positive responses to both systemic and local treatments, which agrees with previous findings [7, 61]. Garcia and Arenas report the successful treatment of a case of *Aspergillus niger*

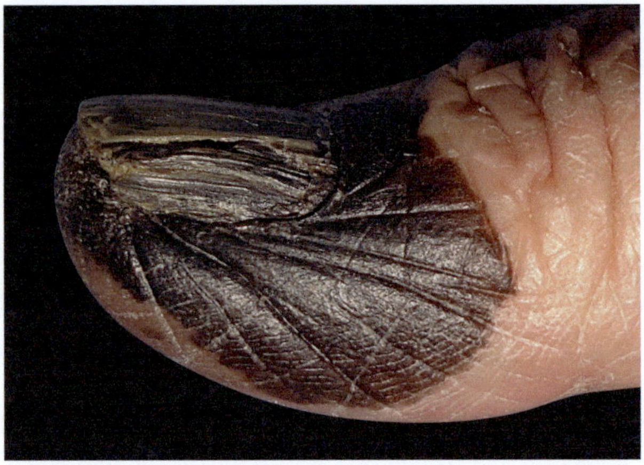

Fig. 9.12 Subungual melanoma, Hutchinson's sign

infection with 2 months of oral terbinafine and topical 1 % bifonazole plus 40 % urea cream [21]. In cases of onychomycosis due to *Alternaria* infection, studies report a favorable response to treatment with itraconazole [28, 62].

Newer antifungal agents include tavaborole, the first FDA-approved oxaborole antifungal agent, and efinaconazole 10 % topical solution, a triazole recently approved for the treatment of onychomycosis [63–65].

Summary for the Clinician

Fungal melanonychia constitutes 1.5–17.5 % of onychomycoses. It is most often caused by opportunistic filamentous pigmented fungi (phaeoids or dematiaceous organisms). Non-dematiaceous causative agents include some dermatophytes, *Candida* and *Aspergillus*. Causative agents have a worldwide distribution.

Ungual infections occur in immunocompetent hosts. Pathogen identification is key to planning adequate treatment, due to the wide variety of possible causative agents and because dematiaceous fungi are resistant to most antifungal drugs.

Differential diagnosis includes diseases that cause non-mycotic melanonychia, mainly frictional melanonychia of the fourth and fifth toes, racial longitudinal melanonychia, and subungual hematomas. Adult-onset melanonychia in particular is an alarming sign that warrants careful investigation in order to rule out melanoma.

Clinical Pearls

Fungal melanonychia presents as dark-brown or black pigmentation of the nail. It can also show dystrophy, onycholysis, nail thickening, and subungual hyperkeratosis, with a distal, lateral, linear, or proximal distribution. It is often accompanied by paronychia. *Candida* and *Neoscytalidium* are the most common pathogens.

Direct examination reveals filaments of irregular thickness that appear to have a double contour.

These fungi do not grow in cycloheximide-containing media. Colonies grow rapidly in culture; colonies of dematiaceous varieties are gray to dark in color.

The treatment of onychomycosis due to non-dermatophytic molds is difficult. In most cases onychomycosis can be cured with chemical or surgical removal of the infected tissues, followed by local antifungal treatment. Some cases required systemic treatment.

Bibliography

1. Finch J, Arenas R, Baran R. Fungal melanonychia. J Am Acad Dermatol. 2012;66:830–41.
2. Arenas R. Micología médica ilustrada. 5th ed. México: McGraw-Hill; 2014. p. 70, 81, 371
3. Odds FC, Arai T, Disalvo AF, et al. Nomenclature of fungal diseases: a report and recommendations from sub-committee of the international society for human and animal mycology (ISHAM). J Med Vet Mycol 1992:30:1–10.
4. Moreno G, Arenas R. Other fungi causing onychomycosis. Clin Dermatol. 2010;28:160–3.
5. Ortega-Springall MF, Arroyo-Escalante S, Arenas R. Onycholysis and chromonychia: A case Caused by *Trichosporoninkin* Skin appendage Disorders 2015;1:144–6.
6. Brandt ME, Warnock DW. Epidemiology, clinical manifestations, and therapy of infections caused by dematiaceous fungi. J Chemother. 2003;15(Suppl 2):36–47.
7. English MP. Nails and fungi. Br J Dermatol. 1976;94:697–701.
8. Tosti A, Piraccini BM, Lorenzi S. Onychomycosis caused by nondermatophytic molds: clinical features and response to treatment of 59 cases. J Am Acad Dermatol. 2000;42:217–24.
9. Woo P, Ngan A, Tsang C, et al. Clinical spectrum of *Exophiala i*nfections and a novel e*xophiala s*pecies, *Exophiala hongkongensis*. J Clin Microbiol. 2013;51(1):260–7.
10. Allison VY, Hay RJ, Campbell CK. *Hendersonula toruloidea* and *Scytalidium hyalinum* infections in Tobago. Br J Dermatol. 1984;111:371–2.
11. Lacroix C, Kac G, Dubertret L, et al. Acytalidios in Paris, France. J Am Acad Dermatol. 2003;48:852–6.
12. Hay RJ, Morre MK. Clinical features of superficial fungal infections caused by *Hendersonula* and *Scytalidium hyalinum*. Br J Dermatol. 1984;110:677–83.
13. Crespo-Erchiga V, Martínez-García S, Martínez-Pilar L. Dermatomicosis por *Scytalidium*. Piel. 2005;20:408–503.
14. Campos P, Arenas R. Melanoniquia fúngica por *Alternaria alternata*. Dermatol Rev Mex. 2013;57:261–3.

15. Arrese JE, Piérard-franchimont C, Piérard-Gerald E. Onychomycosis and keratomycosis caused by *Alternaria* Sp.: a bipolar opportunistic infection in a wood-pulp worker on chronic steroid therapy. Am J Dermatopathol. 1996;18:611–3.
16. Singh SM, Pouranik M. Ungual and cutaneous phaeohyphomycosis caused by *Alternaria alternata* and *Alternaria chlamydospora*. J Med Vet Mycol. 1990;28:275–8.
17. Baxter M. The stimulation of pigment production by *Trichophyton rubrum* on a new medium. Sabouraudia. 1963;3:72–80.
18. Badillet G, Panagiotidou D, Sene S. Etude restrospective des *trichophyton rubrum* á pigment noir diffusible isolés á Paris de 1971 a 1980. Bull Soc Fr Mycol Med. 1984;1:117–20.
19. Youngchim S, Pornsuwan S, Nosanchuk J, et al. Melanogenesis in dermatophyte species *in vitro* and during infection. Microbiology. 2011;157:2348–56.
20. Ray AC, Eakin RE. Studies on the biosynthesis of aspergillin by *Aspergillus niger*. Appl Microbiol. 1975;30:909–15.
21. Tosti A, Piraccini BM. Proximal subungual onychomycosis due to Aspergillus niger: report of 2 cases. Br J Dermatol. 1998;139:156–7.
22. García C, Arenas R, Vasquez del Mercado E. Subungual black onychomycosis and melanonychia striata caused by aspergillus niger. Skinmed. 2015;13:104–6.
23. Parlak AH, Goksugur N, Karabay O. A case of melanonychia due to *Candida albicans*. Clin Dermatol. 2006;31:398–400.
24. Velez A. Melanonychia due to *Candida humícola*. Br J Dermatol. 1996;134:374–5.
25. Gautret P, Rodier MH, Kauffman-Lacroix C, Jacquemkin JL. Case report and review: onychomycosis due to *Candida parapsilosis*. Mycoses. 2000;43:443–5.
26. Lee SW, Kim YC, Kim DK, et al. Fungal melanonychia. J Dermatol. 2004;31:904–9.
27. Morris-Jones R, Gomez BL, Diez S, et al. Synthesis of melanin pigment by *Candida albicans* in vitro and during infection. Infect Immun. 2005;73:6147–50.
28. Seyedmojtaba S, Netea M, Mouton W, et al. Black yeasts and their filamentous relatives: principles of pathogenesis and host defense. Clin Microbiol Rev. 2014;27(3):527–52.
29. Romano C, Paccagnini E, Difonzo EM. Onychomycosis caused by Alternaria spp. in Tuscany, Italy from 1985 to 1999. Mycoses. 2001;44:73–6.
30. Glowacka A, Wasowska-Krolikowska K, Skowron-Kobos J, Kurnatowski M, Janniger CK. Childhood onychomycosis: alternariosis of all ten fingernails. Pediatr Dermatol. 1998;62:125–8.
31. Baran R, Tosti A, Piraccini BM. Uncommon clinical patterns of Fusarium nail infection: report of three cases. Br J Dermatol. 1997;136:424–7.
32. Gupta AK, Ryder JE, Baran R, Summerbell RC. Non-dermatophyte onychomycosis. Dermatol Clin. 2003;21:257–68.
33. Tasić S, Stojanović S, Poljacki M. Etiopathogenesis, clinical picture and diagnosis of onychomycosis. Med Pregl. 2001;54(1–2):45–51.
34. Karaarslan K, Acar A, Aytimur D, Ozdemir F. Dermoscopic features in fungal melanonychia. Clin Exp Dermatol. 2015;40(3):271–8.
35. Piraccini BM, Dika E, Fanti PA. Tips for diagnosis and treatment of nail pigmentation with practical algorithm. Dermatol Clin. 2015;33(2):185–95.
36. Braun RP, Baran R, Le Gal FA, et al. Diagnosis and management of nail pigmentations. J Am Acad Dermatol. 2007;56:835–47.
37. Mun JH, Kim GW, Jwa SW, et al. Dermatoscopy of subungual haemorrhage: its usefulness in differential diagnosis from nail-unit melanoma. Br J Dermatol. 2013;168:1224–9.
38. Taek S, Wong D, Young J, Baik K. Hydroxyurea induced melanonychia concomitant with a dermatomyositis like eruption. J Am Acad Dermatol. 2003;49(2):339–41.
39. Gupta A, Parakh A, Dubey AP. Chemotherapy induced nail changes. Indian J Dermatol. 2008;53(4):204–5.
40. Kumar S, Dixit R, Karmakar S, Paul S. Unusual nail pigmentation following cyclophosphamide containing chemotherapy regimen. Indian J Pharmacol. 2010;42(4):243–4.

41. Chawre SM, Pore S, Nandeshware MB, Masood MN. Zidovudine-induced nail pigmentation in a 12 year old boy. Indian J Pharmacol. 2012;44(6):801–2.
42. Lopez M, Jordao C, Grinszpan R, et al. Chromonychia secondary to chemotherapy. Case Rep Dermatol. 2013;5(2):163–7.
43. Sachdeva S, Sachdeva S, Kapoor P. Laugier-hunziker syndrome: a rare cause of oral and acral pigmentation. J Cutan Aesthet Surg. 2011;4(1):58–60.
44. Wang WM, Wang X, Duan N, et al. Laugier-Hunziker syndrome: a report of three cases and literature review. Int J Oral Sci. 2012;4(4):226–30.
45. Fryer JM, Werth VP. Pregnancy-associated hyperpigmentation: longitudinal melanonychia. J Am Acad Dermatol. 1992;26(3):493–4.
46. Prat C, Viñas M, Marcoval J, Juclá A. Longitudinal melanonychia as the first sign of Addison's disease. J Am Acad Dermatol. 2008;58(3):522–4.
47. Schepis C, Siragusa M, Palazzo R. Multiple melanonychia as a sign of pituitary adenoma. Clin Exp Dermatol. 2013;38:689–90.
48. Juhlin L, Baran R. On longitudinal melanonychia after healing of lichen planus. Acta Derm Venereol. 1990;70:183.
49. Skowron F, Combemale P, Faisant M, et al. Functional melanonychia due to involvement of the nail matrix in systemic lupus erythematosus. J Am Acad Dermatol. 2002;47(Suppl):S187–8.
50. Baran R. Longitudinal melanonychia in localized scleroderma. J Am Acad Dermatol. 2002;50(3):e11–3.
51. Baran R. Longitudinal melanonychia: a symptom of Bowen disease. J Am Acad Dermatol. 1988;18(6):1359–60.
52. Saito T, Uchi H, Moroi Y, et al. Subungual Bowen disease revealed by longitudinal melanonychia. J Am Acad Dermatol. 2012;67(5):e240–1.
53. Sanchez-Carpinteiro I, Belen A, Feito M, et al. Longitudinal melanonychia secondary to a squamous cell carcinoma in situ caused by a papilloma virus infection. J Am Acad Dermatol. 2012;66(4 Suppl 1):AB3.
54. Hernandez C, Elsaady E, Wang S. Pigmented squamous cell carcinoma presenting as melanonychia striata mimicking melanoma. J Am Acad Dermatol. 2015;72(5 Suppl 1):AB189.
55. Rudolph RI. Subungual basal cell carcinoma presenting as longitudinal melanonychia. J Am Acad Dermatol. 1987;16(1 Part 2):229–33.
56. Antonovich DD, Grin C, Grant-Kels JM. Childhood subungual melanoma in situ in diffuse nail melanosis beginning as expanding longitudinal melanonychia. Pediatr Dermatol. 2005;22(3):210–2.
57. Lorizzo M, Tosti A, Di Chiacchio N, et al. Nail melanoma in children. differential diagnosis and management. Dermatol Surg. 2008;34(7):974–8.
58. Tosti S, Piraccini BM, Cagalli A, Haneke E. In situ melanoma of the nail unit in children:report of two cases in fair skinned Caucasian children. Pediatr Dermatol. 2012;29(1):79–84.
59. Levit EK, Kagen MH, Scher RK, et al. The ABC rule for clinical detection of subungual melanoma. J Am Acad Dermatol. 2000;42:269–74.
60. Chabasse D, Pihet M. Onychomycosis due to molds. J Mycol Med. 2014;24(4):261–8.
61. Elewski BE. Onychomycosis caused by *Scytalidium dimidiatum*. J Am Acad Dermatol. 1996;35:338.
62. Gianni C, Romano C. Clinical and histological aspects of toenail onychomycosis caused by *aspergillus* spp: 34 cases treated with weekly intermittent terbinafine. Dermatology. 2004;209:104–10.
63. De Donker PR, Scher RK, Rl B, et al. Itraconazole therapy is effective for pedal onychomycosis caused by some nondermatophyte molds and in mixed infection with dermatophytes and molds: a multicenter study with 36 patients. J Am Acad Dermatol. 1997;36:173–7.
64. Sharma N, Sharma D. An upcoming drug for onychomycosis:Tavaborole. J Pharmacol Pharmacother. 2015;6(4):236–9.
65. Lipner SR, Sher RK. Efinaconazole in the treatment of onychomycosis. Infect Drug Resist. 2015;8:163–72.

Part II
Why and How You Should Confirm Diagnosis

Chapter 10
Direct Microscopy and Culture: What You Need to Know

Roberto Arenas, Diana C. Vega, and Julieta Ruiz-Esmenjaud

Key Features

KOH, chlorazol black, calcofluor white, and culture are the current mycological studies to confirm onychomycosis.

Direct examination in dermatophytic onychomycosis shows septate filaments, arthrospores, or dermatophytoma.

In yeast infections pseudohyphae and blastospores are usually observed.

Onychomycoses are nail infections caused by dermatophytes, yeasts, and non-dermatophytic molds (NDM). Direct examination with KOH, chlorazol black, calcofluor white, and culture are the current mycological studies to confirm the clinical diagnosis [1–4].

Direct examination is performed from the sample obtained by nail scraping with a scalpel blade, a curette, or a vertical perforation of the nail plate [4]. The most convenient site to obtain it, in distal subungual onychomycosis, is from the nail bed or from the ventral area, as well as the proximal part of the affected nail; in the white superficial forms, one scratches the friable part of the dorsal aspect of the nail; in the proximal forms, one must perform a small hole in the proximal part of the nail to expose the affected site of the nail and perform the scraping. In cases of candidal paronychia, one can take small fragments from the cuticle.

This examination is performed with sodium or potassium hydroxide (KOH or NaOH) 10–40% on the nail scraping and slightly heating the sample with a Bunsen lighter, or we can avoid the heating if the KOH is mixed at equal proportions with dimethyl sulfoxide (DMSO). Nowadays, chlorazol black is suitable because it stains just the fungal chitin and is easily observed with a dark or blue color, and artifacts are not confused with fungi structures (Fig. 10.1). If a fluorescence microscope is

R. Arenas (✉) • D.C. Vega • J. Ruiz-Esmenjaud
Mycology Section, Dr. Manuel Gea González General Hospital, México, DF, México
e-mail: rarenas98@hotmail.com; vssdiana@hotmail.com; jwlyetta@hotmail.com

A. Tosti et al. (eds.), *Onychomycosis*, DOI 10.1007/978-3-319-44853-4_10

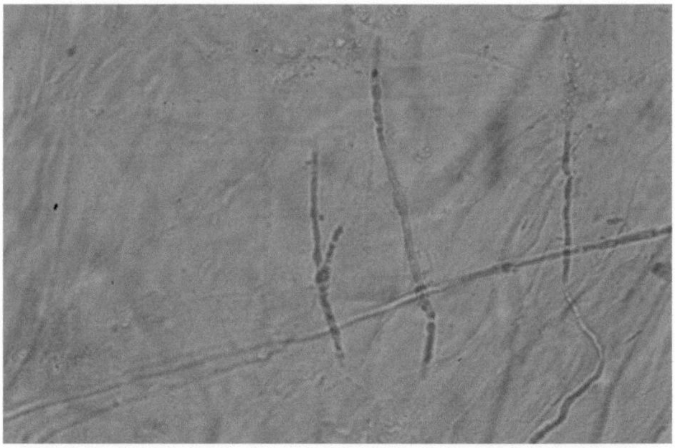

Fig. 10.1 Direct examination in nail clipping (chlorazol black 40×)

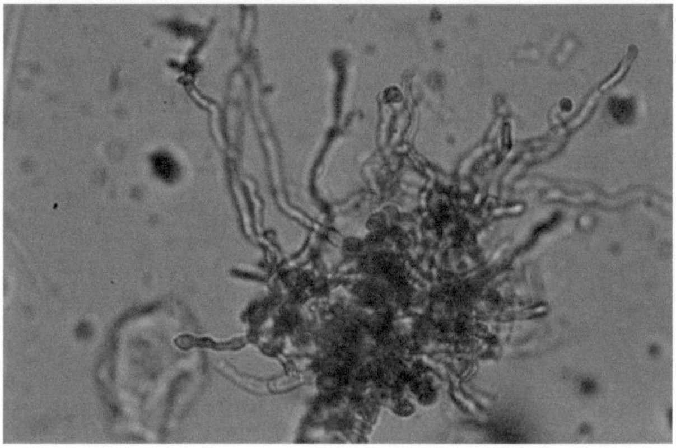

Fig. 10.2 Dermatophytoma (chlorazol black 40x)

available, we can perform the fluorochrome, calcofluor white stain; this is a desirable method, because it allows to visualize even few elements [4, 5].

Long or septate filaments and arthrospores are observed under the microscope. In dermatophytic infection, a dermatophytoma can be found, this is a large accumulation of filaments and spores, and these fungal elements can explain in some cases the lack of response to treatment (Fig. 10.2).

In *Candida* onychomycosis, one can visualize hyphae, pseudohyphae, and blastospores. In dematiaceous fungi we can find dark hyphae, but some non-dermatophytic molds may give similar images to dermatophytes, but in some of them, special characteristics are observed as, in *Aspergillus,* aspergillar heads; in *Scopulariopsis*, huge lemon-shaped spore; and, in *Scytalidium*, narrow and tortuous hyphae [4].

False negatives are due to inexperience in obtaining or reading the sample (20%). Microscopic exam does not allow us to distinguish the viable and nonviable forms [4].

Culture is performed in Sabouraud dextrose agar (SDA) with antibiotics such as chloramphenicol and cycloheximide (Actidione®) if a primary pathogenic fungus is suspected, but the use of culture mediums is convenient without Acti-dione® if

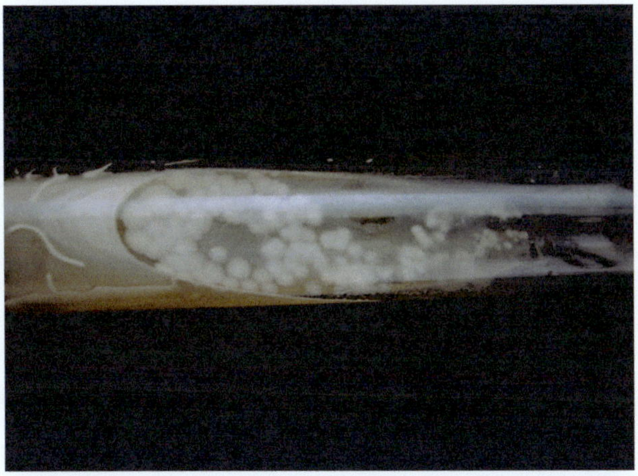

Fig. 10.3 *Candida* spp. culture in SDA

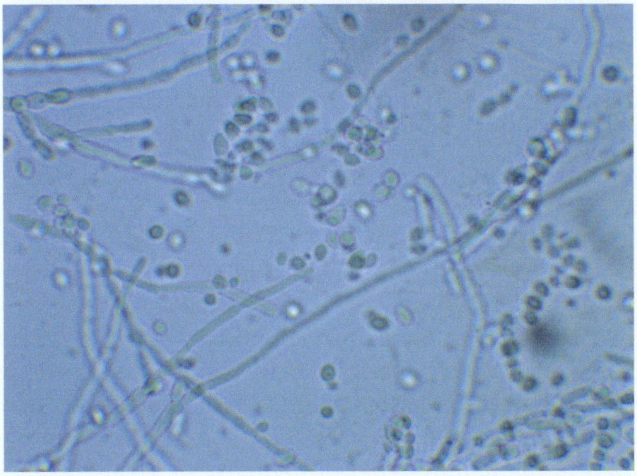

Fig. 10.4 *Candida* spp. blastospores, hyphae, and pseudohyphae

one suspects a non-dermatophytic mold or a yeast (Figs. 10.3 and 10.4). It is convenient to put in the tube or in the Petri dish small fragments of the nail or to pulverize the sample [4].

Usually, it is difficult to isolate the causal agent given the poor sample and the low viability (30–60%); this percentage of false negatives increases after having received a recent treatment or when the scraping is not taken in the limit between the healthy and diseased nail.

Cultures must be incubated at room temperature (24–28° C), and the colonies can be observed from 1 week to 1 month, but NDM and yeasts can grow in less than 1 week; culture is considered negative after 3–6 weeks. If negative, it could be convenient to repeat the complete mycological study [1–4], especially if we have also a negative KOH.

Isolated fungi require a proper interpretation of the mycological samples, because not all the yeasts and non-dermatophytic molds are necessarily pathogens, and should be isolated in several occasions or should grow in abundance in the cultures.

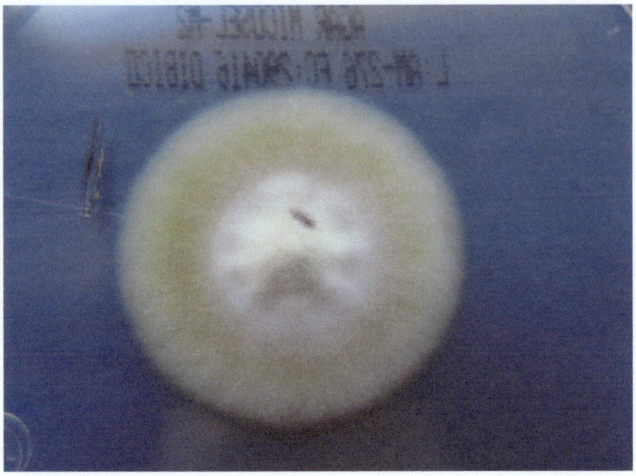

Fig. 10.5 *Trichophyton rubrum*. Culture in SDA

If a specialized personnel is not available, DTM (dermatophyte test medium) is recommended; this is a medium with antibacterial and red phenol as indicators, so bacteria will be inhibited, and if a dermatophyte grows, there is a color virage from yellow to red.

The fungi more frequently isolated among dermatophytes are mainly *Trichophyton rubrum* (Fig. 10.5) and *T. mentagrophytes* var. *interdigitale* and very rare are *T. mentagrophytes* var. *mentagrophytes*, *T. tonsurans*, *Epidermophyton floccosum*, *Microsporum canis, M. gypseum*, *T. soudanense*, *T. violaceum*, *T. erinacei*, and *T. equinum*. Among the yeasts especially *C. albicans* and *C. parapsilosis,* some cases related with *Candida ciferri* and in immunocompromised hosts *Candida glabrata.* Among NDM: *Scopulariopsis brevicaulis* (Fig. 10.6), *Fusarium* sp. and *Aspergillus* sp., *Acremonium* sp., *Paecilomyces* sp., *Onychocola canadensis* Also *Neoscytalidium* sp., *Alternaria alternata, Chaetomium globosum* and another black fungi. It has been informed of lethal dissemination of the infection by *Fusarium* from an onychomycosis in a neutropenic patient [4].

Biopsy is the gold standard, but usually it can be performed when a case of onychomycosis is highly suspicious and the mycological exams are negative or in uncommon cases. A 4 mm punch biopsy can be performed or a longitudinal, and lateral 2 mm biopsy is preferred that includes all the length of the nail, including matrix, proximal fold, nail bed, and hyponychium [5–7].

In onychomycosis, microabscess with leukocytes in the horny layer can be found, spongiosis, leukocytes exostosis, and lymphocytes, sometimes spongiform pustules and the presence of fungi elements in variable quantities.

In lateral and distal subungual onychomycosis, the filaments are visualized in the hyponychium or in the nail bed, and they take a longitudinal distribution; also, round spores can be observed and correspond to dermatophyte arthrospores

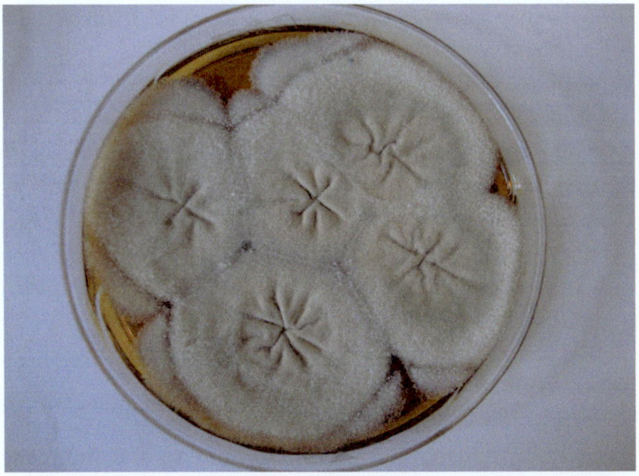

Fig. 10.6 *Scopulariopsis brevicaulis*. Culture in SDA

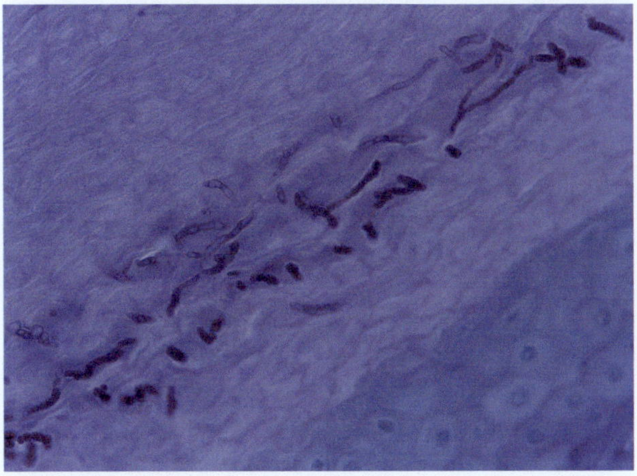

Fig. 10.7 Hyphae and spores (PAS 40×)

(Fig. 10.7); papillomatosis can be present in the nail bed as well as neutrophil microabscesses in the horny layer, spongiosis, and exocytosis; the inflammatory reaction can be mild. In leukonychia cases, the fungi behave as saprophytes with "tortuous" hyphae, arthrospores in chains, short hypha, and even the so-called perforation organs; there is not an inflammatory reaction in the nail bed [4]. In the PWSO a thick lamina is observed with abundant fungal elements and a mild inflammatory reaction. In the total dystrophic onychomycosis, the nail plate is irregular or can lose all its structure. When *Candida* is the causal agent, one can visualize spores and germinated tubes and lymphocyte exocytosis with cerebriform nuclei [4].

In some cases of nail psoriasis, we can find more pronounced parakeratosis, subungual abscesses in the horny layer, spongiform pustules, and parakeratosis foci. Histopathology of the nail allows to differentiate onychomycosis from other inflammatory entities such as lichen planus, alopecia areata, and eczema. Some saprophytic fungi or secondary colonization can mainly affect previously damaged nails [4–7].

The biopsy can be an important diagnostic tool, detecting the fungus using H&E and PAS stains. The histological test with PAS stain is fast, simple, and reliable in evaluating onychodystrophies, and the onychomycosis of the nail plate shows a low sensitivity (62%) but a high specificity (100%); Gomori-Grocott or Gridley [6–8] can be performed and also the KONCPA technique (KOH treated nail clipping stained with PAS) or fluorescence techniques [9].

We can use antibodies, immunohistochemistry, and flow cytometry as other techniques to identify pathogenic fungi in the nail.

In another section of this book, we mention molecular techniques such as PCR to increase sensitivity and specificity of the diagnostic tools. It has been found that the gene fragments that codify for 18S-rARN are amplified in the infected nails, but not in the healthy ones, to be able to recognize the spices and also the RFLP (restriction fragment length polymorphism) patterns, using HaeII endonucleases [10–12].

Summary for the Clinician

Direct examination with KOH, chlorazol black, calcofluor white, and culture are the current mycological studies to confirm clinical diagnosis. It is performed after nail scraping with a scalpel blade or a curette. Chlorazol black is suitable because it stains just the chitin and fungal elements that are easily observed with a dark or blue color.

Causal agents are difficult to isolate, especially dermatophytes (30–60%). Yeasts and NDM must be isolated in a huge quantity.

Biopsy is the gold standard, but it is usually performed when a case of onychomycosis is highly suspicious and the mycological exams are negative.

Molecular tools are also available.

Clinical Pearls

Nail scraping and examination with KOH, chlorazol black, and calcofluor white usually confirm clinical diagnosis of onychomycosis.

Dermatophytes are causal agents which are difficult to isolate. Also yeasts and NDM can be etiological agents.

Biopsy is usually performed when one suspects onychomycosis and mycological exams are negative.

References

1. Haldane DJM, Robart E. A comparison of calcofluor white, potassium hydroxide, and culture for the laboratory diagnosis of superficial fungal infection. Diagn Microbiol Infect Dis. 1990;13:337–9.
2. Bonifaz A, Rios-Yuil JM, Arenas R, et al. Comparison of direct microscopy, culture and calcofluor white for the diagnosis of onychomycosis. Rev Iberoam Micol. 2013;30(2):109–11.
3. RiosYuil JM, Bonifaz A, Arenas R, et al. Mycological studies of nail samples obtained by curettage vs vertical perforation of the nail plate. JEADV. 2012;9:1–2.
4. Arenas R. Métodos diagnósticos nas onicomicosis. In: Di Chiacchio N, Belda Junior W, Criado PR. Unhas. Oque há de novo. Atheneu. São Paul. 2012:11–15.
5. Weinberg JM, Koestenblatt EK, Tutrone WD, Tishler HR, Najarian L. Comparison of diagnostic methods in the evaluation of onychomycosis. J Am Acad Dermatol. 2003;49:193–7.
6. Wilsmann-Theis D, Sareika F, Bieber T, Schmid-Wendtner MH, Wenzel J. New reasons for histopathological nail-clipping examination in the diagnosis of onychomycosis. J Eur Acad Dermatol Venereol. 2011;25(2):235–7.
7. Haneke E. Nail biopsies in onychomycosis. Mykosen. 1985;28:473.
8. Mayer E, Izhak OB, Bergman R. Histopathological periodic acid-schiff stains of nail clippings as a second-line diagnostic tool in onychomycosis. Am J Dermatopathol. 2012;34:270–3.
9. Liu HN, Lee DD, Wong CK. KONCPA: a new method for diagnosing tinea unguium. Dermatology. 1993;187:166–8.
10. Rezaie S, Pourmojib M, Tschacler E. Isolation of total RNA from dermatophytes. Mycoses. 1999;42:615–7.
11. Mochizuki T, Sugie N, Uchara M. Random amplification of polymorphyc DNA is useful for the differentiation of several anthropophilic dermatophytes. Mycoses. 1997;40:405–9.
12. Luk NM, Hui M, Cheng S, Tang LS, Ho KM. Evaluation of PCR for the diagnosis of dermatophytes in nail specimens from patients with suspected onychomycosis. Clin Exp Dermatol. 2012;37:230–4.

Chapter 11
Molecular Techniques (PCR)

Rigoberto Hernández-Castro, Ramón Fernández-Martínez, Gabriela Moreno-Coutiño, and Roberto Arenas

Key Features

- The polymerase chain reaction (PCR) is a highly sensitive and specific molecular technique for onychomycosis diagnosis.
- The commercial kits allow an ideal DNA extraction from clinical samples of onychomycosis and fungal cultures.
- The genomic regions mostly used for onychomycosis diagnosis are the ITS1 and ITS2 region. Other useful genes are the chitin synthase 1 and β-tubulin.
- The panfungal primers are the principal ones for fungal species identification.
- The real-time PCR helps identify fungal presence and its species in clinical samples in a fast and specific way.
- The sequencing of the PCR-amplified DNA is highly sensitive and specific for fungal species identification.

Introduction

The conventional method for the identification of the etiological agents of onychomycosis is the fungal culture, considered the gold standard; however, it has several disadvantages such as a high rate of false-negative results and when it does grow,

R. Hernández-Castro
Department of Ecology of Pathogens Agents, Dr. Manuel Gea González General Hospital, México, DF, México

R. Fernández-Martínez • G. Moreno-Coutiño • R. Arenas (✉)
Mycology Section, Dr. Manuel Gea González General Hospital, México, DF, México
e-mail: rarenas98@hotmail.com

A. Tosti et al. (eds.), *Onychomycosis*, DOI 10.1007/978-3-319-44853-4_11

the utilized time may take up to 4 weeks to do so. These disadvantages are being tried to decrease with the development of molecular techniques that allow species identification in a time span of 24–48 h, which is a considerable reduction when compared to 4 weeks. These techniques also permit the detection of difficult-to-grow fungi and generate reproducible results with high specificity and sensibility.

Although molecular techniques are still not used as routine tests for these purposes, its applications in investigative protocols have been constantly increasing during the last years and, thus, have allowed a cost reduction in its supplies making it more accessible. The downside of molecular biology is that it requires qualified personnel and the specific infrastructure to develop the procedures.

State of the Art

DNA Extraction

DNA extraction is a crucial step for any molecular technique either for basic or clinical research with any microorganism or cell type. The extraction methodology must allow the DNA obtained to be of the highest quality, purity, and integrity. The different methods vary according to the origin of the DNA sample, from a clinical sample or from a pure culture. When working with fungi, specialized techniques are required because of the characteristic components of the fungal cell wall; they can be mechanic, physic, or enzymatic [1–3]. The majority of DNA isolation methods involve three steps: cellular lysis, inactivation of nucleases, and purification.

For DNA extraction by enzymatic digestion (cellular lysis), Proteinase K, lyticase, zymolyase, or other cell wall-degrading enzymes are used [4, 5]. The mechanic procedure includes freezing with liquid nitrogen and crushing of the sample with mortar and pestle, sand, or glass beads. The physical methods may break the cellular wall with microwaves or sonication [6–8]. To obtain a sufficient amount of DNA, these methods require a large quantity of clinical sample and DNA-purifying substances such as phenol-chloroform and RNAse treatment. Something that we must keep in mind is that the physical and mechanical methods may cause DNA rupture or degradation [1–3, 9].

For DNA extraction, the noncommercial methods are very efficient when using a large amount of fungal culture; however, they are not recommended for working with large amounts of clinical samples or paraffin-embedded tissues. The use of commercial methods is very helpful for molecular diagnosis in all sample types and avoids cross contamination, they can handle large number of samples, and the methodological standardization and reagents are simple and faster to use and sometimes even more cost-effective [6, 10–12]. The process includes cellular lysis, RNA removal, protein and polysaccharide elimination, and the union by centrifugation of

DNA to the column. The centrifugation is usually done under refrigeration and requires several wash cycles with tube change in every extraction. The purity, integrity, and amount of DNA obtained are higher than the obtained via noncommercial methods [13–15].

For the reasons mentioned above, the use of commercial kits has increased when fungal DNA extraction is required. Some of the most popular are Fast DNA Kit (Qbiogene, Irvine, CA, USA), ZR Fungal/Bacterial DNA Kit (Zymo Research, Irvine, CA, USA), DNeasy Plant Mini Kit or DNeasy Blood and Tissue DNA Extraction Kits (Qiagen, Valencia, CA, USA), UltraClean Soil DNA Isolation Kit (Mo Bio Laboratories Inc., Carlsbad, CA, USA), MasterPure Yeast DNA Purification Kit (Epicenter, Madison, WI), and High Pure PCR Template Kit (Roche, Basel, Switzerland) among others. All the commercial extraction systems share the use of columns.

Molecular Techniques

The development and application of molecular techniques have increased during the last decades with the purpose to improve the sensitivity and/or specificity of diagnosis, as well as to decrease the periods of time normally required for detection and identification of etiological agents.

In clinical samples from patients with onychomycosis, several strategies are used based on the DNA detection for dermatophytes and non-dermatophytes. The classic technique is the polymerase chain reaction (PCR).

Polymerase Chain Reaction (PCR)

The polymerase chain reaction (PCR) is a molecular technique widely used to make multiple copies of a specific gene or gene fragments.

This molecular tool is very precise and can be used to amplify or copy a specific DNA target from a mixture of DNA molecules in vitro, where the DNA polymerase enzyme synthetizes a complementary sequence of DNA using two short DNA sequences called primers, free nucleotides, MgCl2, and nucleotides (A, T, C, G); the mixture is placed in a PCR machine, called thermocycler. The chain reaction involves a process of exponential amplification: one DNA molecule is used to produce two copies of specific fragment and then four, then eight, and then millions of copies [16]. Despite that one of the most important characteristics of PCR is its high sensitivity, it can produce false-positive results due to exogenous contamination. To avoid this, some strategies must prevail such as physical separation of work areas: DNA extraction area, PCR area, and electrophoresis area.

A classic PCR is called end point PCR, which may be uniplex or simple, multiplex, and nested. Also, this can be combined with other techniques such as restriction fragment length polymorphism analysis (PCR-RFLP), where restriction enzymes that recognize specific sites in the material obtained by PCR generate fragments with different lengths which conform patterns unique to each species of dermatophyte or non-dermatophyte involved. Direct sequencing to the product obtained by PCR has proven to be a great technique for species or subspecies identification. PCR may be used in a real-time protocol (PCR real time) with the intention to quantify the relative levels of the transcription of the genetic marker of choice and to estimate the viability of the sample. Although PCR has the advantage of consuming much less time than fungal culture, it has the disadvantage of being a more expensive technique, particularly the PCR sequencing or PCR real time [17–28].

Gene Target

For gene target options, the internal transcribed spacer regions ITS1 and ITS2 are the gene region most commonly used for sequencing and identifying a large number of fungi. They are variable regions located between the conserved genes that codify for the ribosomal subunits 18S, 5.8S, and 28S.

Ribosomal DNA (rDNA) is a tandem region of 50–100 copies in the fungal haploid genome. It is composed of the gene of the small subunit (SSU) rDNA (18S), the gene from subunit 5.8S, and the gene from the large subunit (LSU) rDNA (28S). When separating the subunits 18S and 5.8S, and subunits 5.8S and 28S, we find the intergenic transcribed spacers (ITS), ITS1 and ITS2, respectively (Fig. 11.1). Besides this cluster, we find a second repeated unit of the gene of the subunit 5S rDNA flanked by a region of the non-transcribed spacer (NTS). Either cluster can be used as a marker for PCR. The genes in the subunits of rDNA are highly conserved and the ITS regions are highly variable among fungi [29].

The region ITS1 can be amplified from a wide variety of fungus by using the primers ITS1 (5-TCCGTAGGTGAACCTTGCGG-3) and ITS2 (5-GCTGCGTTCTTCATCGATGC-3). A second variable zoned among the cluster

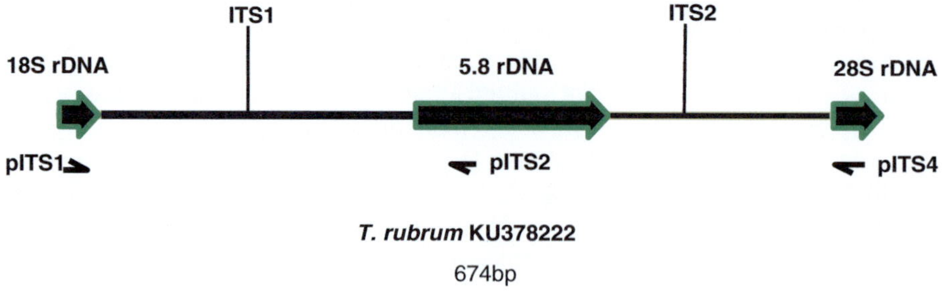

Fig. 11.1 Map of rDNA locus from *Trichophyton rubrum*

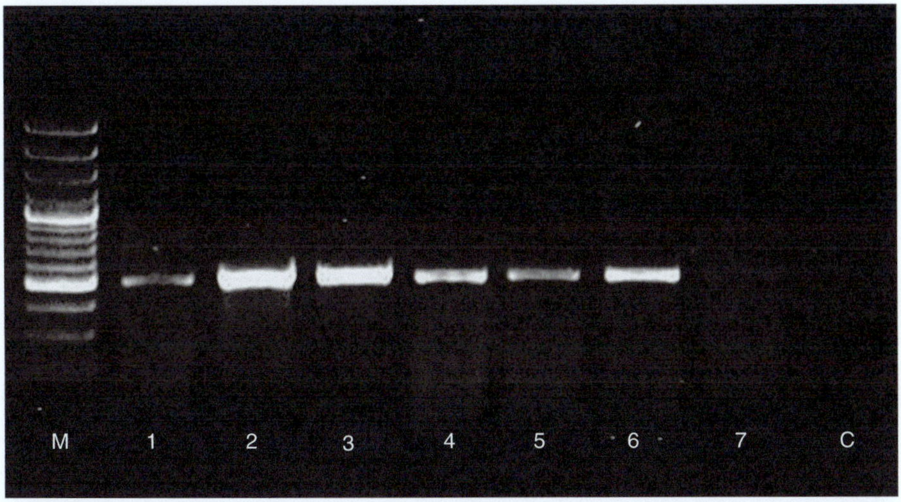

Fig. 11.2 The 18S-ITS1-5.8S-ITS2-28S rDNA amplification using the ITS1 and ITS4 primers of *Trichophyton rubrum* from nail samples. M, 100 bp DNA ladder; line 1, *T. rubrum* positive control; lines 2–7, DNA from nails with onychomycosis; C, negative control

of ribosomal DNA has an area named domain D1/D2, located in the rDNA 28S subunit. This region can be amplified with ITS1 primers (5-TCCGTAGGT GAACCTTGCGG-3) and ITS4 (5-TCCTCCGCTTATTGATATGC-3) (Fig. 11.2). They are highly conserved and informative and much less variable than the ITS. The conserved region of the domains D1/D2 is the anchorage point for the primers that, along with the variable nature of the ITS regions, provides a specific combination for each species. One of the main advantages of the ribosomal locus in fungi is the high number of copies from the target gene, 10–100 times, compared to genes with only one copy, what in the end translates in higher sensitivity [11, 19, 22, 30–33].

A gene frequently used is the chitin synthase 1 (CHS1), and in cases where the ribosomal target is not sensitive enough for discriminating between closely related species, additional loci may be sequenced, such as the β-tubulin [11, 19, 22, 30–33].

More recently, real-time PCR (quantitative PCR [qPCR]) has been used to identify onychomycosis, using molecular beacons which are small single-chain probes of hairpin type that fluoresce when linked to the target site. The same way as with conventional PCR (end point PCR), both variable and conserved regions (ITS1-2/ITS1-4) can be used to design the probe. This will allow the universal identification of the fungal presence in the sample or the involved species [34].

On the other hand, in the same qPCR platform, TaqMan technology or hybrid probes can be used, such as the carboxyfluorescein (FAM)-labeled probe with a Black Hole Quencher (BHQ1) [35, 36]. This technique can detect and quantify quickly the nucleic acids directly from human and animal tissue samples. It has high sensitivity with a detection threshold of one single molecule and depends from one efficient DNA extraction and purification to avoid PCR inhibitors as well as an adequate fungal cell wall lysis [11, 12].

Panfungal Amplification Technique

The gene regions in the SSU and the LSU rDNA have highly conserved regions and variable regions [31, 37]. These permit the development of panfungal primers based on the conserved regions of the rRNA cluster which are capable of identifying a great number of fungal species and can even be species specific [27, 29, 31]. These characteristics have made this the preferred PCR mode. After the amplification of the mentioned region, different genders and species can be identified using the same amplification product by RFLP, hybridization with specific probes marked with radioactivity or digoxigenin, and, with highly specific tool, the direct sequencing of the amplification product [38–41].

A general problem with PCR as detection method for the causative agents of onychomycosis is the lack of worldwide standardization, as well as the deficit of availability of commercial systems in some countries. Several studies report excellent results with "in-house PCR"; however, the majority of these don't make adequate comparisons mainly in clinical practice [22, 42]. The DNA extraction methods, genetic markers, as well as the different types of clinical samples (blood, DNA from fungal culture, nails, the hair, the skin, or fluids) are factors that influence the comparison between different PCR protocols.

Outlook: Future Developments

Molecular biology is a tool under continuous development and improvement for onychomycosis diagnosis.

The challenges ahead are:

- Availability of molecular tests to reduce the time consumed in some techniques such as PCR sequencing, corroborate sensitivity, and specificity of the currently available tests and improve them if possible with the aim to reduce the clinical sample required that at present must be large
- Improvement of keratin extraction and fungal cell wall rupture techniques
- Reduction of costs
- Readily accessible kits for fast etiological identification in onychomycosis, particularly when caused by non-dermatophyte molds or yeasts, which enables the indication of adequate treatment options
- Improvement of subspecies identification
- More than one fungal determination in the same clinical sample
- Differentiation of saprophytes from etiological agents
- Performance of epidemiological studies to redefine onychomycosis frequency and its etiological agents
- Implementation of matrix-assisted laser desorption/ionization time-of-flight mass spectrometry (MALDI-TOFMS) in clinical samples

- Identification of the species of causative agents with PCR-terminal restriction fragment length polymorphism (PCR-TRFLP)
- Implementation of the use of other operons as genes that codify for non-ribosomal proteins and determine if relapses are by the same causative agent

Summary for the Clinician
Molecular techniques are particularly useful for fast identification of onychomycosis in atypical or mycological negative cases, gender and species identification in 24–48 h allowing a prompt diagnosis, and thus optimal management.

Clinical Pearls
Consider molecular biology for diagnosis in difficult onychomycosis cases:
- Identify fungal genus and species in onychomycosis if traditional techniques have failed to do so.
- Send enough of the clinical sample for adequate processing.
- Contact a reference center that has access to molecular biology for difficult onychomycosis cases.

References

1. Manian S, Sreenivasaprasad S, Mills PR. DNA extraction method for PCR in mycorrhizal fungi. Lett Appl Microbiol. 2001;33(4):307–10.
2. Karakousis A, Tan L, Ellis D, Alexiou H, Wormald PJ. An assessment of the efficiency of fungal DNA extraction methods for maximizing the detection of medically important fungi using PCR. J Microbiol Methods. 2006;65(1):38–48.
3. Sasidharan K, Amariei C, Tomita M, Murray DB. Rapid DNA, RNA and protein extraction protocols optimized for slow continuously growing yeast cultures. Yeast. 2012;29(8):311–22.
4. Ling M, Merante F, Robinson BH. A rapid and reliable DNA preparation method for screening a large number of yeast clones by polymerase chain reaction. Nucleic Acids Res. 1995;23(23):4924–5.
5. Williamson EC, Leeming JP, Palmer HM, Steward CG, Warnock D, Marks DI, Millar MR. Diagnosis of invasive aspergillosis in bone marrow transplant recipients by polymerase chain reaction. Br J Haematol. 2000;108(1):132–9.
6. van Burik JA, Schreckhise RW, White TC, Bowden RA, Myerson D. Comparison of six extraction techniques for isolation of DNA from filamentous fungi. Med Mycol. 1998;36(5):299–303.
7. Velegraki A, Kambouris M, Kostourou A, Chalevelakis G, Legakis NJ. Rapid extraction of fungal DNA from clinical samples for PCR amplification. Med Mycol. 1999;37(1):69–73.
8. Lurá MC, Benitez JD, Jáuregui S, González AM. Evaluación de diferentes técnicas de extracción del ADN de hongos filamentosos. Revista FABICIB. 2003;7:37–44.
9. Romanelli AM, Fu J, Herrera ML, Wickes BL. A universal DNA extraction and PCR amplification method for fungal rDNA sequence-based identification. Mycoses. 2014;57(10):612–22.

10. Haugland RA, Heckman JL, Wymer LJ. Evaluation of different methods for the extraction of DNA from fungal conidia by quantitative competitive PCR analysis. J Microbiol Methods. 1999;37(2):165–76.
11. Chen SC, Halliday CL, Meyer W. A review of nucleic acid-based diagnostic tests for systemic mycoses with an emphasis on polymerase chain reaction-based assays. Med Mycol. 2002;40(4):333–57.
12. Fredricks DN, Smith C, Meier A. Comparison of six DNA extraction methods for recovery of fungal DNA as assessed by quantitative PCR. J Clin Microbiol. 2005;43(10):5122–8.
13. Rittenour WR, Park JH, Cox-Ganser JM, Beezhold DH, Green BJ. Comparison of DNA extraction methodologies used for assessing fungal diversity via ITS sequencing. J Environ Monit. 2012;14(13):766–74.
14. Vesper S. Traditional mould analysis compared to a DNA-based method of mould analysis. Crit Rev Microbiol. 2011;37(1):15–24.
15. Keswani J, Kashon ML, Chen BT. Evaluation of interference to conventional and real-time PCR for detection and quantification of fungi in dust. J Environ Monit. 2005;7(4):311–8.
16. Clark D, Pazdernik NJ. Fundaments of the polymerase chain reaction. In: Clark D, Pazdernik NJ, editors. Molecular biology. 2nd ed. Oxford: Elsevier Inc.; 2013. p. 163–93.
17. Hall L, Wohlfiel S, Roberts GD. Experience with the MicroSeq D2 large-subunit ribosomal DNA sequencing kit for identification of filamentous fungi encountered in the clinical laboratory. J Clin Microbiol. 2004;42(2):622–6.
18. Gupta AK, Simpson FC. Diagnosing onychomycosis. Clin Dermatol. 2013;31(5):540–3.
19. Gräser Y, Czaika V, Ohst T. Diagnostic PCR of dermatophytes: an overview. J Dtsch Dermatol Ges. 2012;10:721–5.
20. El Fari M, Tietz HJ, Presber W, Sterry W, Gräser Y. Development of an oligonucleotide probe specific for *Trichophyton rubrum*. Br J Dermatol. 1999;141(2):240–5.
21. Kano R, Nakamura Y, Watanabe S, Tsujimoto H, Hasegawa A. Phylogenetic relation of *Epidermophyton floccosum* to the species of *Microsporum* and *Trichophyton* in chitin synthase 1 (CHS1) gene sequences. Mycopathologia. 1999;146(3):111–3.
22. Brillowska-Dabrowska A, Saunte DM, Arendrup MC. Five-hour diagnosis of dermatophyte nail infections with specific detection of *Trichophyton rubrum*. J Clin Microbiol. 2007;45(4):1200–4.
23. Garg J, Tilak R, Singh S, Gulati AK, Garg A, Prakash P, Nath G. Evaluation of pan-dermatophyte nested PCR in diagnosis of onychomycosis. J Clin Microbiol. 2007;45(10):3443–5.
24. Ebihara M, Makimura K, Sato K, Abe S, Tsuboi R. Molecular detection of dermatophytes and nondermatophytes in onychomycosis by nested polymerase chain reaction based on 28S ribosomal RNA gene sequences. Br J Dermatol. 2009;161(5):1038–44.
25. Uchida T, Makimura K, Ishihara K, Goto H, Tajiri Y, Okuma M, et al. Comparative study of direct polymerase chain reaction, microscopic examination and culture-based morphological methods for detection and identification of dermatophytes in nail and skin samples. J Dermatol. 2009;36(4):202–8.
26. Litz CE, Cavagnolo RZ. Polymerase chain reaction in the diagnosis of onychomycosis: a large, single-institute study. Br J Dermatol. 2010;163(3):511–4.
27. de Assis SD, de Carvalho Araújo RA, Kohler LM, Machado-Pinto J, Hamdan JS, Cisalpino PS. Molecular typing and antifungal susceptibility of *Trichophyton rubrum* isolates from patients with onychomycosis pre- and post-treatment. Int J Antimicrob Agents. 2007;29(5):563–9.
28. Arabatzis M, Bruijnesteijn van Coppenraet LE, Kuijper EJ, de Hoog GS, Lavrijsen AP, Templeton K, et al. Diagnosis of common dermatophyte infections by a novel multiplex real-time polymerase chain reaction detection/identification scheme. Br J Dermatol. 2007;157(4):681–9.
29. Reiss E, Tanaka K, Bruker G, Chazalet V, Debeaupuis JP, Hanazawa R, et al. Molecular diagnosis and epidemiology of fungal infections. Med Mycol. 1998;36(Suppl 1):249–57.

30. Kan VL. Polymerase chain reaction for the diagnosis of candidaemia. J Infect Dis. 1993;168(3):779–83.
31. White TJ, Bruns T, Lee S, Taylor J. Amplification and direct sequencing of fungal ribosomal RNA genes for phylogenetics. In: Innis MA, Delfand DH, Sninsky JJ, White TJ, editors. PCR protocols. San Diego: Academic Press; 1990. p. 315–22.
32. Faergemann J, Baran R. Epidemiology, clinical presentation and diagnosis of onychomycosis. Br J Dermatol. 2003;149(Suppl 65):1–4.
33. Jensen RH, Arendrup MC. Molecular diagnosis of dermatophyte infections. Curr Opin Infect Dis. 2012;25(2):126–34.
34. Park S, Wong M, Marras SA, Cross EW, Kiehn TE, Chaturvedi V, et al. Rapid identification of *Candida dubliniensis* using a species-specific molecular beacon. J Clin Microbiol. 2000;38(8):2829–36.
35. Tyagi S, Kramer FR. Molecular beacons: probes that fluoresce upon hybridisation. Nat Biotechnol. 1996;14(3):303–8.
36. Brandt M, Padhye A, Mayer LW, Holloway BP. Utility of random amplified polymorphic DNA PCR and TaqMan automated detection in molecular identification of *Aspergillus fumigatus*. J Clin Microbiol. 1998;36(7):2057–62.
37. Kappe R, Fauser C, Okeke CN, Maiwald M. Universal fungus-specific primer systems and group-specific hybridisation oligonucleotides for 18S rDNA. Mycoses. 1996;39(1–2):25–30.
38. Medlin L, Elwood HJ, Stickel S, Sogin ML. The characterization of enzymatically amplified eukaryotic 16-S like rRNA-coding regions. Gene. 1988;71(2):491–9.
39. Hopfer RL, Walden P, Setterquist S, Highmith WE. Detection and differentiation of fungi in clinical specimens using polymerase chain reaction (PCR) amplification and restriction enzyme analysis. J Med Vet Mycol. 1993;31(1):65–75.
40. Einsele H, Hebart H, Roller G, Löffler J, Rothenhofer I, Müller CA, et al. Detection and identification of fungal pathogens in blood by using molecular probes. J Clin Microbiol. 1997;35(6):1353–60.
41. Van Burik JA, Myerson D, Schreckhise RW, Bowden RA. Panfungal PCR assay for the detection of fungal infection in human blood specimens. J Clin Microbiol. 1998;36(5):1169–75.
42. Nenoff P, Krüger C, Schaller J, Ginter-Hanselmayer G, Schulte-Beerbühl R, Tietz HJ. Mycology-an update Part 2: dermatomycoses: clinical picture and diagnostic. J Dtsch Dermatol Ges. 2014;12(9):749–77.

Chapter 12
Onychomycosis: Role of Histopathology

Paola Flores-Gavilán, Sonia Toussaint-Caire, and Roberto Arenas

> **Key Features**
> - Histopathological examination of nail clippings is the most sensitive technique for onychomycosis diagnosis.
> - Special stains like periodic acid-Schiff (PAS) and Grocott methenamine silver (GMS) are required to highlight the presence of fungal hyphae.
> - The infecting agent can be suspected depending on its exposed architecture; nevertheless, the precise identification is not possible.

Onychomycosis is the term used to describe fungal infection of one or more nail units, caused primarily by dermatophytes, yeasts, or non-dermatophyte molds (NDM). It represents the most frequent onychopathy in adults, accounting for up to 50 % of all nail disorders and affecting approximately 5–13 % of the general population, proportionately increasing with age [1, 2]. Clinical presentation can be variable and may mimic other nail diseases so diagnostic tests need to be conducted to confirm the presence of fungi [3].

Traditionally, onychomycosis is diagnosed by two standard methods, direct examination with KOH-Chlorazol black® (Delasco, Council Bluffs) and fungal culture; nevertheless, inconsistent low sensitivities of these techniques have been reported, resulting in potentially delayed diagnosis, which may lead to total nail dystrophy, with low rates of recovery despite treatment [2, 4]. Thus, histopathological examination can be useful when the latter are negative and can be helpful in

P. Flores-Gavilán, MD • S. Toussaint-Caire, MD
Dermatology Division, Dermatopathology Section, Dr. Manuel Gea González General Hospital, México, DF, México

R. Arenas (✉)
Mycology Section, Dr. Manuel Gea González General Hospital, México, DF, México
e-mail: rarenas98@hotmail.com

A. Tosti et al. (eds.), *Onychomycosis*, DOI 10.1007/978-3-319-44853-4_12

establishing the extent of the fungal invasion, suggesting an infective agent or ruling out the infection by proposing an alternative diagnosis [2, 5].

The infected nail is clinically and histopathologically different from the healthy nail. Electron microscopy has been useful in characterizing the microscopic nail plate architecture in normal and affected nails. Healthy nails have a smooth surface made of parallel layers of flat and keratinized cells called onychocytes, resulting in a compact barrier; they have an average reported thickness of 0.49 mm and a density of 1.34 g/cm^3. On the other side, onychomycotic nails present a fragmented surface with cell separation and lifting, indicating its rigidity has changed; also, they tend to be thicker (1.29 mm) and have a lower density (1.29 g/cm^3) than non-affected nails, traducing a more porous plate [5, 6].

Dermatophytes are known to have a variety of proteases and lipases that hydrolyze keratin, collagen, and elastin, which alter the nail matrix, disrupt cell interactions, and help them invade the nail plate, so explaining the reported microscopic changes [7, 8].

The most frequent type of nail biopsy for diagnosing onychomycosis is the nail clipping dyed with special fungal stains, which is now considered the gold standard because of its high sensitivity. This is the preferred diagnostic method because it is a non-painful procedure for the patient and is fast and simple to perform at a low cost.

Clippings are fragments cut from the distal portion of the nail plate, which according to reports should be at least 4 mm in length to improve the diagnostic performance; these samples are then processed and stained for histopathological assessment [9, 10].

With hematoxylin and eosin (HE) stain, the study frequently reveals dystrophy of the nail plate with dissociated keratin layers (Fig. 12.1), as well as the presence of parakeratosis and plasma globules, which according to several studies are statistically and significantly more common in slides where fungi are found than in those where they are not present. Neutrophils and bacteria are variably described; nevertheless, their finding is not statistically different with the presence or absence of fungi. All these microscopic findings are more frequent and easily found on the ventral part of the nail plate, which is in close proximity to the nail bed. In a white superficial onychomycosis, fungal elements are commonly found in the dorsal surface of the nail plate [10, 11].

The fungal hyphae on HE routinely stained sections are difficult to visualize; therefore, special fungi stains are needed to highlight its presence; these classically include periodic acid-Schiff (PAS) and Grocott methenamine silver (GMS). PAS technique works by exposing tissue to periodic acid, which oxidizes hydroxyl groups of cell wall polysaccharides into dialdehydes; the latter react with Schiff reagent, forming a magenta compound. The background is a faint pink, while fungi cell membranes stain a magenta-red color. In GMS stain, chromic acid is used to oxidize the hydroxyl groups forming aldehydes, which then react with the silver nitrate reducing it to metallic silver, making them visible. The slide has a light green background, while the hyphae are stained dark brown to black [1].

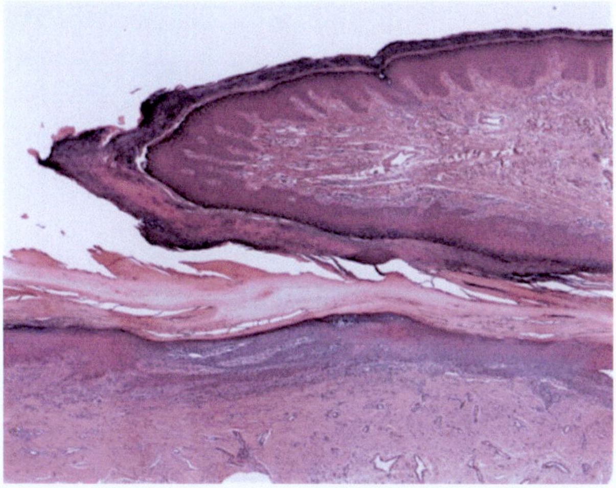

Fig. 12.1 Longitudinal nail biopsy of an onychomycotic nail. The nail plate of the matrix and proximal nail bed is dystrophic showing an irregular, fragmented, and lifted surface with mounds of parakeratosis

For a while, GMS was thought to be superior to PAS staining for finding fungal structures in biopsies; however, after several conducted studies, they concluded the deeper levels were increasing the detection of the fungi, rather than the stain used. Although no significant differences were reported between these two, PAS was found to be a more cost-effective stain [1, 2, 12].

Although the fungi structures are well visualized with the special stains described, histological examination does not allow the precise identification of the infecting agent; however, it can suggest the implicated pathogen by analyzing their morphology.

Usually, a dermatophytic infection is suspected when regular, septate hyphae running parallel to the nail surface are observed (Fig. 12.2).

Yeasts are suspected when small round spores, some even budding, pseudohyphae, and short filaments are found. Spores without pseudohyphae can be contaminants (Fig. 12.3).

NDM can display truncated spores with vertically thin arising perforating hyphae.

Although the former are the main causative onychomycosis agents, other ND fungi have been reported to cause infection like *Aspergillus* spp., *Alternaria* spp., *Scopulariopsis brevicaulis*, *Emericella quadrilineata*, and other microorganisms like *Prototheca* spp., and also Medlar bodies have been found in a case of melanonychia [13–17].

An uncommon and unique clinical presentation of onychomycosis caused by dermatophytes, also known as dermatophytoma, typically presents as a yellow longitudinal band or yellow or white patch. Histologically a dense mass of hyphae is found [10].

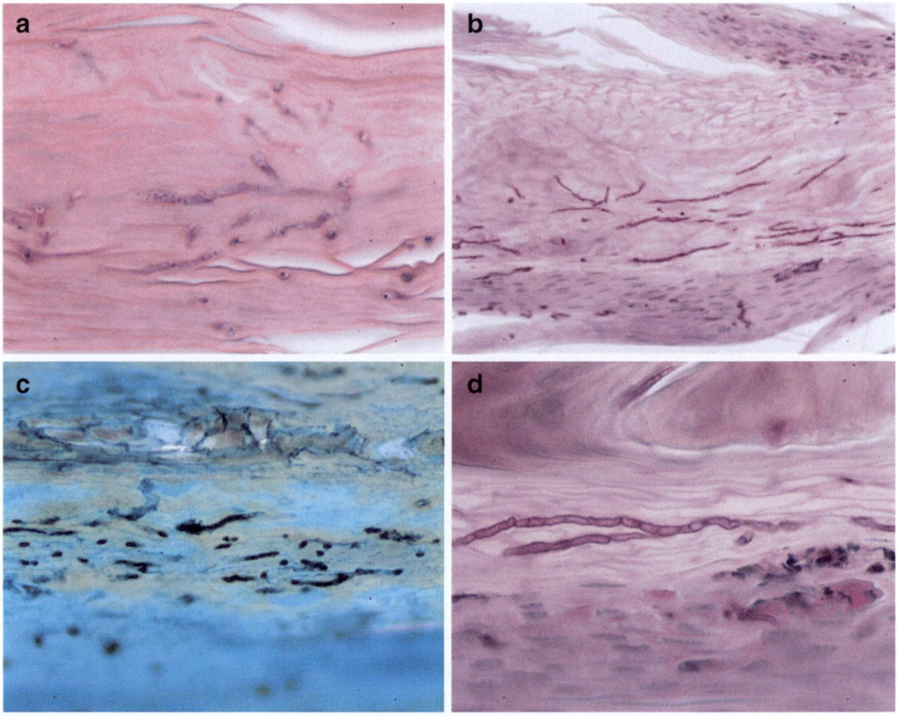

Fig. 12.2 Histological examination of dermatophytic onychomycosis. (**a**) H&E stain showing translucent hyphae spreading between corneocytes. (**b**) PAS stain highlighting hyphae in *red-magenta* color. These are regular and parallel-oriented to the nail surface. (**c**) Hyphae dyed in *black* with Grocott methenamine silver stain. (**d**) PAS stain showing regular, branching, septate hyphae

Punch samples of nail plate and nail bed or longitudinal nail biopsies are rarely performed, except when other inflammatory diseases are clinically suspected. When these are taken, the histological picture displays subungual hyperkeratosis with mounds of parakeratosis or foci of neutrophils, psoriasiform dermatitis with hyperplasia of the nail bed epithelium, and variable spongiosis with neutrophil exocytosis. In the absence of onychomycosis, another nail disorder can be recalled like psoriasis, lichen planus, or even a hematoma. Psoriasis can be difficult to differentiate from onychomycosis clinically and histopathologically [5].

KOH has a sensitivity between 53 and 76 % and mycological culture between 35 and 53 %; both tend to be sample dependent; nevertheless, the latter can identify the fungal species and sensitivities to antifungals but requires long incubation periods to yield a diagnosis. PAS-stained sections of nail clippings have the highest reported sensitivity, varying between 75 and 92 % according to different studies, and therefore are considered the gold standard diagnostic technique. It is the least likely to be affected by sampling methods and is also considered the most sensitive to monitor residual infection after adequate antifungal treatment. Combining these techniques has established decreased chances of false negatives; PAS staining combined with KOH reported sensitivities between 89 and 99.4 %, while PAS with culture gave

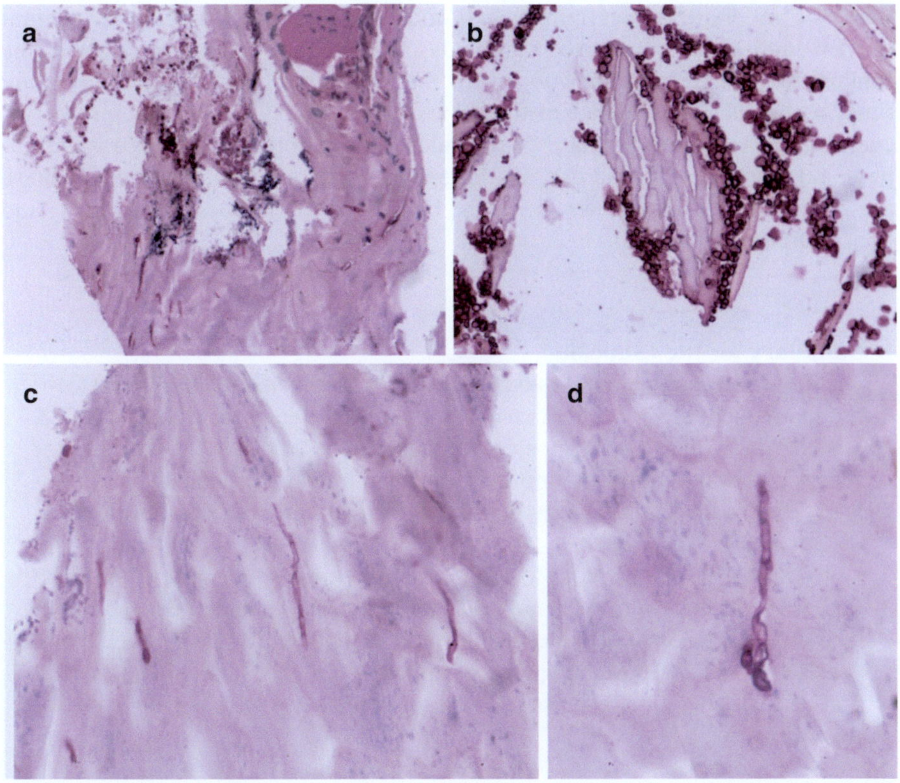

Fig. 12.3 *Candida* onychomycosis on a histological section stained with H&E. (**a**) Dystrophic nail plate with parakeratosis, plasma, bacterial colonies, and *red-magenta* dyed spores. (**b**) Multiple small round spores admixed with keratin. (**c**, **d**) Short and thin filaments and pseudohyphae, vertically oriented to the nail plate, are also found

between 93 and 96 %; however, PAS alone was better than the combination of KOH direct microscopy and culture with a sensitivity of 88.8 %. Hence, combination of PAS-stained nail clippings with either KOH or culture can give higher values of sensitivity and negative predictive values [4, 11, 18].

Although histopathology is a relatively fast diagnostic test, the nail needs to be fixed, dehydrated, embedded in paraffin, and sectioned before being stained [3]. A nail biopsy can be technically harder to process than a routine cutaneous specimen because of the hard keratin in the nail plate, so pretreatment with softening agents is needed to obtain high-quality sections. Useful softener agents described include potassium hydroxide (KOH), 4 % phenol, 5 % trichloroacetic acid in 10 % formalin, cider oil, chitin softening agent with mercuric chloride containing solutions, and more recently sodium hydroxide (NaOH), which has reported an improved ease of sectioning and adherence to slides, although fainter PAS staining and damage to melanin and hemosiderin pigments have been reported [10, 19].

More novel techniques have been described for detecting dermatophytes, for example, fluorescence microscopy, from the basis that some pathogenic fungi fluoresce under ultraviolet light, as in Wood's lamp test. This method uses hematoxylin- and eosin-stained sections under fluorescence microscopy, where the fungus shows a clear bright fluorescent ring at the periphery, without investing time in special stains. Other available tests are flow cytometry, immunohistochemistry, phase-contrast hard X-ray microscopy, optical coherence tomography, and DNA-based rapid diagnostic techniques like PCR; nevertheless, these are limited and infeasible for daily use because of high costs, complexity, and poor availability [18, 20].

Summary for the Clinician

Histological examination of nail clippings is a simple and relatively fast technique for diagnosing onychomycosis. Sections typically need PAS or GMS stains to highlight the presence of hyphae. PAS nail clipping has the highest reported sensitivity and, therefore, is considered the gold standard; nevertheless, combination with KOH or mycological culture is recommended to enhance diagnostic yield.

Histological examination does not allow the precise identification of the fungal agent; however, it can suggest the implicated pathogen depending on its morphology. Dermatophytes display regular septate hyphae parallel to nail surface; yeasts show round spores, pseudohyphae, and short filaments; and non-dermatophyte molds present with truncated spores with thin and vertical perforating hyphae.

Clinical Pearls

- PAS staining of nail clippings is the gold standard for diagnosing onychomycosis. This is usually performed when KOH or mycological culture yields negative results and clinical suspicion is high.
- Morphology of fungi can suggest the etiological pathogen.
- When a longitudinal nail biopsy is performed, it displays subungual hyperkeratosis with mounds of parakeratosis or foci of neutrophils, psoriasiform hyperplasia of the nail bed epithelium, and variable spongiosis with neutrophil exocytosis.
- Nail biopsies allow other nail disorders to be excluded. Psoriasis is the principal differential diagnosis.
- Although it is relatively simple and fast technique, nail biopsy can be technically harder to process.
- Combination of diagnostic tests is recommended to improve diagnostic performance.

References

1. Barak O, Asarch A, Horn T. PAS is optimal for diagnosing onychomycosis. J Cutan Pathol. 2010;37:1038–40.
2. Reza Kermanshahi T, Rhatigan R. Comparison between PAS and GMS stains for the diagnosis of onychomycosis. J Cutan Pathol. 2010;37:1041–4.
3. Gupta A, Simpson FC. Diagnosing onychomycosis. Clin Dermatol. 2013;31:540–3.
4. Jeelani S, Ahmed QM, Lanker AM, Hassan I, Jeelani N, Fazili T. Histopathological examination of nail clippings using PAS staining (HPE-PAS): gold standard in diagnosis of Onychomycosis. Mycoses. 2015;58:27–32.
5. André J, Sass U, Richert B, Theunis A. Nail pathology. Clin Dermatol. 2013;31:526–39.
6. Baraldi A, Jones SA, Guesné S, Traynor MJ, McAuley WJ, Brown MB, Murdan S. Human nail plate modifications induced by onychomycosis: implications for topical therapy. Pharm Res. 2015;32:1626–33.
7. Monod M. Secreted proteases from dermatophytes. Mycopathologia. 2008;166:285–94.
8. Hellgren L, Vincent J. Lipolytic activity of some dermatophytes. II. Isolation and characterisation of the lipase of *Epidermophyton floccosum*. J Med Microbiol. 1981;14(3):347–50.
9. Neto JF, Tchornobay AM. How the nail clipping helps the dermatologist. An Bras Dermatol. 2009;84(2):173–6.
10. Stephen S, Tosti A, Rubin AI. Diagnostic applications of nail clippings. Dermatol Clin. 2015;33:289–301.
11. Mayer E, Izhak OB, Bergman R. Histopathological periodic acid–schiff stains of nail clippings as a second-line diagnostic tool in onychomycosis. Am J Dermatopathol. 2012;34:270–3.
12. D'Hue Z, Perkins SM, Billings SD. GMS is superior to PAS for diagnosis of onychomycosis. J Cutan Pathol. 2008;35:745–7.
13. Arrese JE, Piérard-Franchimont C, Piérard C. Onychomycosis and keratomycosis caused by *Alternaria* sp. A bipolar opportunistic infection in a wood-pulp worker on chronic steroid therapy. Am J Dermatopathol. 1996;18(6):611–3.
14. Stefanato CM, Verdolini R. Histopathologic evidence of the nondermatophytic mould *Scopulariopsis brevicaulis* masking the presence of dermatophytes in a toenail infection. J Cutan Pathol. 2009;36(Suppl 1):8–12.
15. Sharma D, Capoor MR, Ramesh V, Gupta S, Shivaprakash MR, Chakrabarti A. A rare case of onychomycosis caused by *Emericella quadrilineata* (*Aspergillus tetrazonus*). Indian J Med Microbiol. 2015;33:314–6.
16. Ko CJ, Sarantopoulos GP, Pai G, Binder SW. Longitudinal melanonychia of the toenails with presence of Medlar bodies on biopsy. J Cutan Pathol. 2005;32:63–5.
17. Gandham NR, Vyawahare CR, Chadhaury N, Shinde RA. Onychoprotothecosis: an uncommon presentation of protothecosis. Indian J Med Microbiol. 2015;33:435–7.
18. Stewart CL, Rubin AI. Update: nail unit dermatopathology. Dermatol Ther. 2012;25:551–68.
19. Nazarian RM, Due B, Deshpande A, Duncan LM, Misdraji J. An improved method for surgical pathology testing for onychomycosis. J Am Acad Dermatol. 2012;66(4):655–60.
20. Estela Cubells JR, Victoria Martínez AM, Martínez Leboráns L, Alegre de Miquel V. Fluorescence microscopy as a diagnostic tool for dermatophytosis. Am J Dermatopathol. 2016;38(3):208–10.

Chapter 13
Dermoscopy

Miriam America Jesus-Silva, Rodrigo Roldan-Marin, Daniel Asz-Sigall, and Roberto Arenas

Key Features

- Dermoscopy is a noninvasive tool that has proven to be an important adjunctive in the evaluation of nail diseases.
- Distinctive dermoscopic features for onychomycosis have been reported and include jagged proximal edge with spikes of the onycholytic area, longitudinal striae, and longitudinal or homogenous melanonychia.
  - The "jagged proximal edge area" is never linear and has sharp structures (spikes) with matte pigmentation.
  - The "longitudinal striae pattern" is observed more frequently in patients with TDO or DLSO.
  - The presence of a "linear edge" excludes onychomycosis and suggests traumatic onycholysis.
  - In fungal longitudinal melanonychia, the band of pigmentation is wider distally and narrows proximally.

M.A. Jesus-Silva
Clínica de Onco-Dermatología, Facultad de Medicina. UNAM, Universidad Nacional Autónoma de México, Avenida Universidad 3000, Universidad Nacional Autónoma de México, Mexico City, Mexico

R. Roldan-Marin
Faculty of Medicine, Universidad Nacional Autonoma de Mexico, Circuito Escolar s/n, Anexo 1 Facultad de Medicine, Ciudad Universitaria, Entre Div. Gral CCH and Services Medicos VI, Mexico City, Mexico

D. Asz-Sigall • R. Arenas (✉)
Mycology Section, Dr. Manuel Gea González General Hospital, México, DF, México
e-mail: rarenas98@hotmail.com

A. Tosti et al. (eds.), *Onychomycosis*, DOI 10.1007/978-3-319-44853-4_13

Introduction

Onychopathies are known to be among the most frequent complaints in dermatological practice, either as manifestations of primary diseases or in association with other systemic pathologies. Among these, onychomycosis is one of the most common nail disorders accounting for nearly 50 % of them. Within skin diseases, it has a prevalence of 0.44 % with a worldwide prevalence ranging from 2 to 50 % [1]. It mainly affects adults between 30 and 60 years of age.

The differential diagnosis of onychomycosis includes inflammatory diseases such as psoriasis, lupus erythematosus, lichen planus, lichen striatum, alopecia areata, and pityriasis rubra pilaris and also systemic diseases (amyloidosis, diabetes mellitus, porphyria, dysthyroidism). Infectious diseases that may mimic onychomycosis include viral warts and chronic paronychia. Other important differential diagnoses are cosmetic trauma (manicure or pedicure), secondary trauma (tight shoes or friction), and nail apparatus tumors (squamous cell carcinoma, melanoma, or digital fibroma) [2].

Accurate diagnosis is important since the treatment of onychomycosis can be long-standing and expensive and may be accompanied by severe adverse effects [2]. Currently, the diagnosis is made by clinical suspicion along with potassium hydroxide (KOH) examination followed by culture of the sample [3, 4].

KOH examination and fungal cultures have a sensitivity and specificity ranging between 72–80 % and 72–76 % for KOH and 20–53 % and 82–100 % for fungal cultures that may vary significantly when performed by an experienced mycologist with proper sampling technique [5, 6]. Nail scrapings obtained at the distal part of the nail are often positive for fungal and bacterial contaminants present in the "gateway" of the nail lesion left behind by the real pathogen. Therefore, it is known that sampling for mycological examination should be performed at the most proximal portion of the nail lesion, where there is a higher probability to find the fungus responsible for the nail invasion. However, it may be uncomfortable and even painful for the patient because it requires progression of instruments under the nail plate [6].

Dermoscopy is a noninvasive tool that is widely used for the diagnosis of melanocytic and nonmelanocytic lesions and inflammatory and infectious diseases. It has recently been used as a noninvasive diagnostic tool for the assessment of onychomycosis [7–9].

Epidemiology

Onychomycosis is a common problem in dermatology practice that can result in significant morbidity. Onychomycosis is a chronic fungal infection of the nail and may involve the nail bed, nail plate, and nail matrix. It is difficult to treat and relapses, and reinfections are common [10, 11]. This nail disease may be caused by dermatophytes, yeasts, and nondermatophyte molds [12–15]. Surveys suggest that overall the incidence is much higher in adults than in children, afflicting 0.6 % of children under the age of 18 years, approximately 10–20 % of adults, and 15–40 % of elderly people. The incidence and prevalence of onychomycosis vary from 2 to 4 % in the general population in the United States of America, reaching up to 13 % among Finnish men [16]. The incidence increases with age and nearly 30 % of patients are older than 60 years. Although infrequent, this infection can affect children and is most likely due to the use of occlusive footwear [17]. Some of the contributing risk factors causing this disease are humidity, occlusive footwear, repeated nail trauma, genetic predisposition, and concurrent disease, such as tinea pedis, diabetes mellitus, obesity, peripheral vascular disease (PVD), and HIV infection, as well as other forms of immune suppression [18]. Significant associations also exist for psoriasis [19, 20]. These conditions may contribute to onychomycosis susceptibility via slower/poor nail growth (due to age or poor circulation), suboptimal immune function, and/or nail trauma (diabetic neuropathy, psoriatic nail changes). Vasoconstriction and/or hypoxemia due to nicotine exposure or PVD may further increase the risk of onychomycosis.

Most onychomycoses are caused by dermatophytes that belong to three genera: *Trichophyton*, *Microsporum*, and *Epidermophyton*. Several fungi can be causative agents, but three species predominate worldwide: *T. rubrum*, *T. mentagrophytes*, and *E. floccosum*. *T. rubrum* is found in 60–80 % of cases, *T. mentagrophytes* in 20 %, and *E. floccosum* in 10 % [21–25]. The rest originate from nondermatophyte molds such as *Scopulariopsis* and *Neoscytalidium hyalinum* (formerly *Scytalidium*). *T. rubrum* and *T. mentagrophytes* are the first and second most frequent etiologic agents worldwide [26]. *Candida* spp. are the most frequent among the yeasts.

Clinical Features

There are different clinical subtypes of onychomycosis depending on the degree of affliction.

Distal lateral subungual onychomycosis (DLSO) It is the most frequent type; it affects mainly the hyponychium and side edges, extending proximally and causing subungual hyperkeratosis [27, 28]. The fungus invades proximally and migrates through the underlying nail matrix [27, 29]. There is mild inflammation resulting in parakeratosis and subungual hyperkeratosis, generating onycholysis and thickening of the subungual region with changes in the color of the nail plate secondary to superinfection of bacteria and molds [27].

Superficial white onychomycosis It is much less common than the DLSO; it affects the surface of the nail, not the nail bed [28]. Total destruction of the nail is rarely seen, but the fungus may move through the nail plate and infect the cornified layer of the nail bed and hyponychium [27]. Clinically it is characterized by well-defined opaque “white islands” of the external plate; it is also important to notice that the nail becomes rough, soft, and crumbly [27, 28]. The most frequent site of invasion is the toenail. This subtype can be seen in patients with immunosuppression (AIDS) or in young children with thin toeplates [29].

Subungual and proximal onychomycosis (SPO) It affects the proximal matrix of the nail, and it can be accompanied by paronychia if the infective agent is *Candida* spp. [29]. In this type of onychomycosis, it is important to rule out any cause of immunosuppression since it is not a common subtype. This occurs when the fungus invades the nail unit via the proximal nail fold through the cuticle area, penetrating the new nail plate and migrating distally [27]. Subungual hyperkeratosis, proximal onycholysis, leukonychia, and destruction of the nail plate can be seen [28]. In the case of SPO with paronychia secondary to *Candida* infection, opaque strips of onycholysis along the lateral edges of the nail plate can be seen [28, 29].

Total dystrophic onychomycosis It is characterized by total destruction of the nail plate [27, 28]. There are two main forms: secondary total dystrophic onychomycosis due to the complete progression of any of the different types of onychomycosis and primary total dystrophic onychomycosis due to chronic mucocutaneous candidiasis; in this case, all the tissues of the nail apparatus can be involved simultaneously [29].

Fungal melanonychia It is characterized by brown to black pigmentation of the nail unit; it can be accompanied by a dystrophic and raised plate, secondary to subungual hyperkeratosis. It is common to observe periungual inflammation [30]. The fungal melanonychia can be longitudinal (*T. rubrum* var. *nigricans*) or diffuse brown pigmentation (*Neoscytalidium dimidiatum*, *Aspergillus niger*). In the case of longitudinal melanonychia, the band of pigmentation is wider distally and tapers proximally (distal to proximal extension of infection). There is also a variant of the superficial white onychomycosis that can be referred to as superficial black onychomycosis, commonly caused by *Aspergillus niger* and frequently accompanied by periungual inflammation and black pigmentation of the proximal nail fold [30].

Diagnostic Clues

The use of dermoscopy for the study of nail disorders is recent. In the beginning it was mainly used for the study of nail pigmentations, but now several studies have demonstrated its utility in various nail disorders including onychomycosis [1, 31].

The study should include the proximal nail fold and the hyponychium, and to improve the adherence of the lens to the surface, ultrasound gel should be used, especially when studying melanonychia. To study the nail plate surface, the ultrasound gel should be removed as it can cover surface abnormalities [31].

The main utility of dermoscopy in onychomycosis is to differentiate it from traumatic onycholysis [1] or from true melanonychia [32].

There are three dermoscopic findings that are exclusive for onychomycosis: jagged proximal edge with spikes of the onycholytic area [8], longitudinal striae, and distal irregular termination (ruin appearance) [9, 33]:

- *Jagged proximal edge with spikes of the onycholytic area*: in this pattern the proximal margin of the onycholytic area has a jagged edge, with sharp longitudinal whitish indentations directed to the proximal nail fold (spikes). This pattern is best observed with magnification of 20x [8, 9] and is characteristic of total dystrophic onychomycosis and distal lateral subungual onychomycosis [8] (Fig. 13.1). The spikes correspond to the onset of fungal invasion starting from the low adherence region [8, 33].
- *Longitudinal striae*: also known as "aurora borealis pattern" [8]; in this pattern, different colors of striae can be observed in the onycholytic nail plate; the colors range from white to yellow, orange, and brown and are the reflection of the color of the colonies, scales, and subungual debris and their progression along the nail plate [8, 9] (Fig. 13.2). This pattern is best observed with magnification of 40x [8] and is characteristic of patients with distal lateral subungual onychomycosis.
- *Distal irregular termination or ruin appearance*: this pattern is characterized by indentate areas on the ventral portion of the nail, forming a keratosis aspect that corresponds to the accumulation of dermal debris and distal pulverization characteristic of the thickening of the nail plate in total dystrophic onychomycosis (Fig. 13.3). The absence of clinical distal subungual longitudinal striae is explained by the advanced level of fungal invasion.

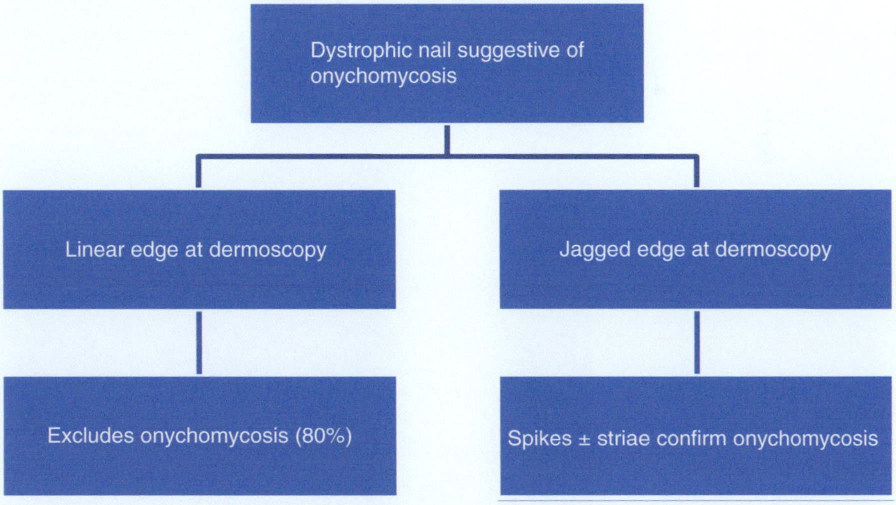

In the case of fungal melanonychia, the most frequent dermoscopic finding can be homogeneous pigmentation (brown, gray, or black) which presents as pigmented lines or structureless discoloration (Fig. 13.4); black pigment aggregates can also be seen and can be coarse granules (matte black, roundish structures >0.1 mm) or

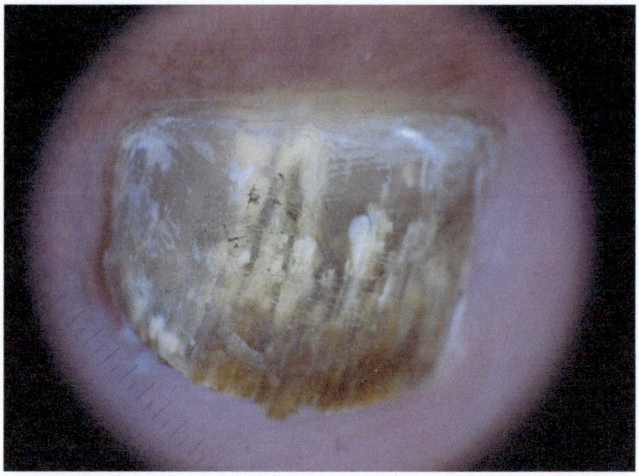

Fig. 13.1 Jagged proximal edge with spikes of the onycholytic area: spiked pattern, indentations at the proximal edge of the area with onycholysis

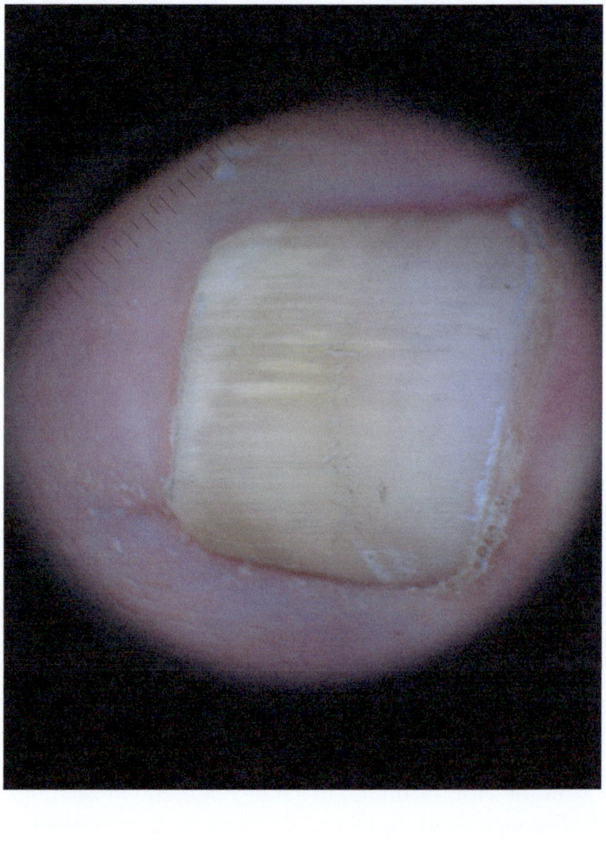

Fig. 13.2 Longitudinal striae. Longitudinal striae of different colors in the onycholytic nail plate

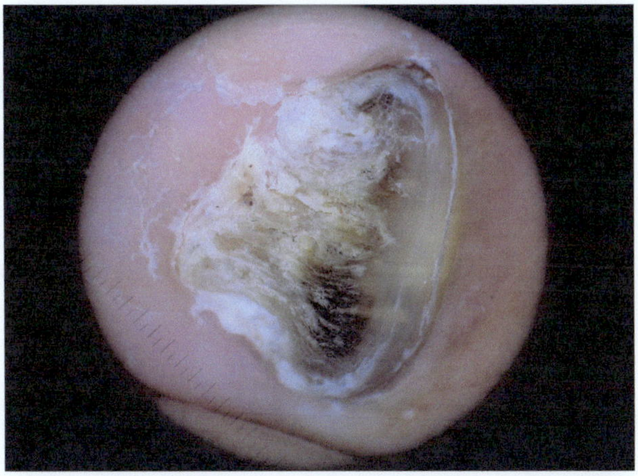

Fig. 13.3 Distal irregular termination or ruin appearance: distal pulverization characteristic of the thickening of the nail plate

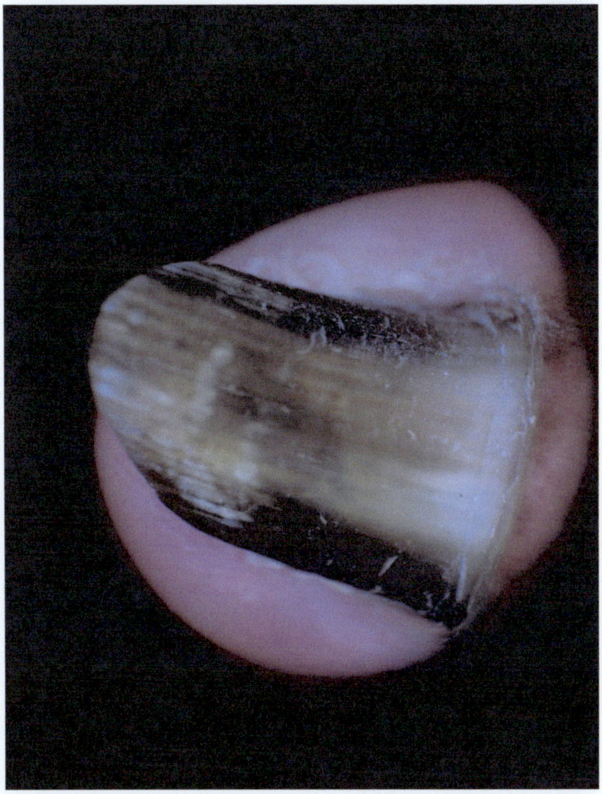

Fig. 13.4 Melanonychia. Homogeneous pigmentation (*black*) structures and pigmented clumps forming larger and irregular shaped structures with different colors

pigmented clumps (aggregated multiple coarse granules forming larger and irregular-shaped structures) [32].

Other dermoscopic features for differentiating fungal melanonychia from other conditions include [32]:

- Multicolored pigmentation (yellow, brown, gray, black or red)
- Matte black pigmentation (lines, disrupted black linear pigmentation or homogeneous areas)
- Black pigment aggregates (coarse granules or pigment clumps)
- Black reverse triangle (wider distally and narrows proximally)
- Superficial transverse striation
- Blurred appearance

It is important to notice that the coarse granules and pigment clumps correlate with the accumulation of fungal colonies and the pigment produced by the fungi, seen in histopathological samples [32].

Summary for the Clinician

Onychomycosis is one of the most common nail disorders (50 % cases). Accurate diagnosis is important since the treatment can be long-standing and expensive and may be accompanied by severe adverse effects. The diagnosis is made by clinical suspicion along with potassium hydroxide (KOH) examination followed by culture of the sample. This method may be uncomfortable and even painful for the patient and may vary significantly when performed by an experienced mycologist with proper sampling technique. Dermoscopy is a noninvasive tool recently used for the study of nail disorders and helpful to differentiate onychomycosis from traumatic onycholysis or true melanonychia. There are three dermoscopic findings exclusive for onychomycosis: jagged proximal edge with spikes of the onycholytic area, longitudinal striae, and distal irregular termination (ruin appearance). In fungal melanonychia the most frequent dermoscopic findings are homogeneous pigmentation (brown, black, or gray) and black pigment aggregates (coarse granules or pigmented clumps). In fungal longitudinal melanonychia, the band of pigmentation is wider distally and narrows proximally.

Clinical Pearls

Dermoscopy is a noninvasive method that helps to differentiate onychomycosis from traumatic onycholysis or true melanonychia.

There are three dermoscopic findings exclusive for onychomycosis:

(a) Jagged proximal edge with spikes of the onycholytic area (characteristic of TDO and DLSO)
(b) Longitudinal striae ("aurora borealis pattern" and characteristic of DLSO)
(c) Distal irregular termination (ruin appearance) seen in TDO

Fungal melanonychia shows homogeneous or longitudinal pigmentation with black pigment aggregates.

References

1. Nakamura RC, Costa MC. Dermatoscopic findings in the most frequent onychopathies: descriptive analysis of 500 cases. Int J Dermatol. 2012;51:483–96.
2. Allevato MA. Diseases mimicking onychomycosis. Clin Dermatol. 2010;28:164–77.
3. Richert B, Lateur N, Theunis A, et al. New tools in nail disorders. Semin Cutan Med Surg. 2009;28:44–8.
4. Harvey CK, Richardson A. Techniques for obtaining specimens for culture to confirm onychomycosis. J Am Podiatr Med Assoc. 2000;90:394–6.
5. Weinberg JM, Koestenblatt EK, Tutrone WD, Tishler HR, Najarian L. Comparison of diagnostic methods in the evaluation of onychomycosis. J Am Acad Dermatol. 2003;49:193–7.
6. Bet DL, dos Reis AL, Di Chiacchio N, Belda JW. Dermoscopy and Onychomycosis: guided nail abrasion for mycological samples. An Bras Dermatol. 2015;90:904–6.
7. Micali G, Lacarrubba F, Massimino D, et al. Dermatoscopy: alternative uses in daily clinical practice. J Am Acad Dermatol. 2011;64:1135–46.
8. Piraccini BM, Balestri R, Starance M, Rech G. Nail digital dermoscopy (onychoscopy) in the diagnosis of onychomycosis. J Eur Acad Dermatol Venereol. 2013;27:509–13.
9. Jesús-Silva MA, Fernández Martínez R, Roldán-Marín R, Arenas R. Dermoscopic patterns in patients with a clinical diagnosis of onychomycosis—results of a prospective study including data of potassium hydroxide (KOH) and culture examination. Dermatol Pract Concept. 2015;5(2):5.
10. Sigurgeirsson B, Olafsson JH, Steinsson JB, Paul C, Billets S, Evans EG. Long-term effectiveness of treatment with terbinafine vs. itraconazole in onychomycosis: a 5-year blinded prospective follow-up study. Arch Dermatol. 2002;138:353–7.
11. Shuster S, Baran R. Recurrence of fungal nail disease and the dissociation of relapse from reinfection. Acta Derm Venereol. 2001;81:154–5.
12. Welsh O, Vera-Cabrera L, Welsh E. Onychomycosis. Clin Dermatol. 2010;28:151–9.
13. Thomas J, Jacobson GA, Narkowicz CK, Peterson GM, Burnet H, Sharpe C. Toenail onychomycosis: an important global disease burden. J Clin Pharm Ther. 2010;35:497–519.
14. Mayser P, Freund V, Budihardja D. Toenail onychomycosis in diabetic patients: issues and management. Am J Clin Dermatol. 2009;10:211–20.
15. Surjushe A, Kamath R, Oberai C, et al. A clinical and mycological study of onychomycosis in HIV infection. Indian J Dermatol Venereol Leprol. 2007;73:397–401.
16. Heikkilä H, Stubb S. The prevalence of onychomycosis in Finland. Br J Dermatol. 1995;133:699–703.
17. Lateur N, Mortaki A, André J. Two hundred ninety-six cases of onychomycosis in children and teenagers: a 10-year laboratory survey. Pediatr Dermatol. 2003;20:385–8.
18. Westerberg DP, Voyack MJ. Onychomycosis: current trends in diagnosis and treatment. Am Fam Physician. 2013;88:762–70.
19. Klaassen KMG, Dulak MG, van de Kerkhof PCM, Pasch MC. The prevalence of onychomycosis in psoriatic patients: a systematic review. J Eur Acad Dermatol Venereol. 2014;28:533–41.
20. Rizzo D, Alaimo R, Tilotta G, Dinotta F, Bongiorno MR. Incidence of onychomycosis among psoriatic patients with nail involvement: a descriptive study. Mycoses. 2013;56:498–9.
21. Effendy I, Lecha M, Feuilhade de Chauvin M, Di Chiacchio N, Baran R, European Onychomycosis Observatory. Epidemiology and clinical classification of onychomycosis. J Eur Acad Dermatol Venereol. 2005;19(Suppl 1):8–12.
22. Hay R. Literature review. Onychomycosis. J Eur Acad Dermatol Venereol. 2005;19(Suppl 1):1–7.
23. Welsh O, Welsh E, Ocampo-Candiani J, Gomez M, Vera-Cabrera L. Dermatophytoses in Monterrey, México. Mycoses. 2006;49:119–23.
24. Seebacher C, Bouchara JP, Mignon B. Updates on the epidemiology of dermatophyte infections. Mycopathologia. 2008;166:335–52.
25. Kaur R, Kashyap B, Bhalla P. Onychomycosis—epidemiology, diagnosis and management. Indian J Med Microbiol. 2008;26:108–16.
26. Gupta AK, Drummond-Main C, Cooper EA, Brintnell W, Piraccini BM, Tosti A. Systematic review of nondermatophyte mold onychomycosis: diagnosis, clinical types, epidemiology, and treatment. J Am Acad Dermatol. 2012;66:494–502.

27. Elewski B. Onychomycosis: pathogenesis, diagnosis and management. Clin Microbiol Rev. 1998;11(3):415–29.
28. Ballesté R, Mousqués N, Gezuele E. Onicomicosis. Revisión del tema Rev Med Urug. 2003; 19:93–106.
29. Baran R, Hay RJ, Tosti A. A new classification of onychomycosis. Br J Dermatol. 1998; 139:567–71.
30. Finch J, Arenas R, Baran R. Fungal melanonychia. J Am Acad Dermatol. 2011; 66(5):830–41.
31. Piraccini B, Bruni F, Starace M. Dermoscopy of non-cancer nail disorders. Dermatol Ther. 2012;25:594–602.
32. Karaarslan K, Acar A, Aytimur D, et al. Dermoscopic features in fungal melanonychia. Clin Exp Dermatol. 2015;40:271–8.
33. Crignis G, Valgas N. Dermatoscopy of onychomycosis. Int J Dermatol. 2014;53:80–1.

Chapter 14
Mimickers

Emilie Fowler and Antonella Tosti

Key Features

- Various nail disorders causing subungual hyperkeratosis and/or onycholysis can mimic onychomycosis.
- Diagnosis of onychomycosis requires laboratory studies.
- Differential diagnosis depends on the clinical type of onychomycosis

Introduction

Onychomycosis is the diagnosis for onychodystrophic nails about 50 % of the time [1]. However, there are a variety of other etiologies that may be causing the onychodystrophic nails. These other conditions may mimic onychomycosis in their presentations and must be excluded before initiating antifungal treatment.

Mimickers for onychomycosis include inflammatory, infective, and neoplastic nail disorders, as well as nail manifestations of systemic diseases. This chapter will discuss differential diagnoses according to the clinical type of onychomycosis.

E. Fowler • A. Tosti, MD (✉)
University of Miami, Department of Dermatology and Cutaneous Surgery, Miami, FL, USA
e-mail: atosti@med.miami.edu

A. Tosti et al. (eds.), *Onychomycosis*, DOI 10.1007/978-3-319-44853-4_14

Distal Subungual Onychomycosis

Differential diagnosis includes nail diseases that cause subungual hyperkeratosis and/or onycholysis.

Subungual hyperkeratosis and onycholysis	Psoriasis
	Contact dermatitis
	Nail bed lichen planus
Onycholysis	Traumas
	Yellow nail syndrome
	Nail bed tumors (warts, exostosis, squamous cell carcinoma, melanoma)
Subungual hyperkeratosis	Pachyonychia congenita

Nail Psoriasis

Epidemiology

Psoriasis of the nails is the most common mimicker of onychomycosis [2]. Psoriasis involves the nails in 80–90 % of patients. Only 5 % of psoriasis cases will have isolated involvement of the nails [1].

Clinical Features

Nail psoriasis presents clinically with pitting, onycholysis with erythematous border, salmon patches, subungual hyperkeratosis, and splinter hemorrhages, among other nail abnormalities [3].

The most common change seen in nail psoriasis is pitting, in which small depressions of less than 1 millimeter diameter are seen on the surface of the nail plate, due to the presence of parakeratotic cells [3]. This is the result of psoriatic lesions, which consist of clusters of parakeratotic cells in the proximal nail matrix. These clusters disrupt normal keratinization and eventually are removed as the nail grows outward, leaving depressions on the nail surface (Fig. 14.1).

A salmon-colored patch may be seen beneath the nail plate, resembling an oil drop. The red-yellow discoloration is the result of parakeratotic lesions within the nail bed that are visible through the overlying nail plate. This “oil drop” sign is the most diagnostic finding of nail psoriasis. Onycholysis occurs when the parakeratotic lesions involve the hyponychium. Air enters the space between the nail bed and overlying nail plate and may cause white discoloration [1]. Psoriatic onycholysis is typically surrounded by an erythematous border.

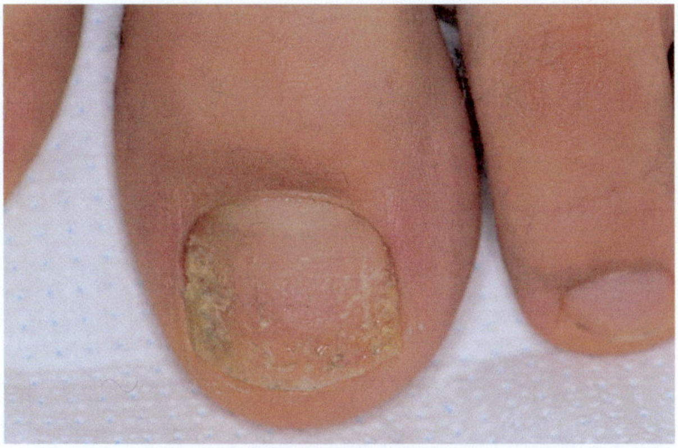

Fig. 14.1 Nail psoriasis. The presence of pitting suggests diagnosis

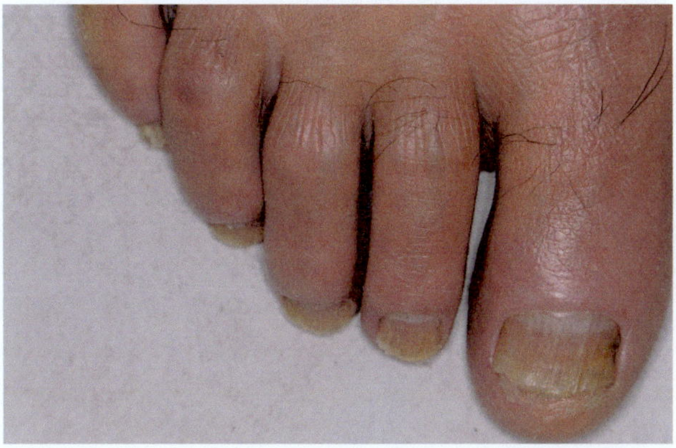

Fig. 14.2 Nail psoriasis presenting with subungual hyperkeratosis, onycholysis, and yellow discoloration

Subungual hyperkeratosis results from deposition and accumulation of desquamated cells underneath the nail plate. This leads to detachment of the nail plate from the nail bed. The degree of this detachment depends upon the level of psoriatic activity present. Subungual hyperkeratosis in nail psoriasis is typically characterized by a silvery-white discoloration as opposed to the typical yellow, greasy appearance seen in onychomycosis, but this is not always the case [1, 4] (Fig. 14.2).

Splinter hemorrhages are less commonly seen and appear as linear, thin, deep, red to black lines in the distal nail. These occur in the dermis of the nail bed, when small capillaries rupture into the linearly oriented epidermal-dermal ridges. Splinter hemorrhages are not only associated with psoriasis, as they can present in a number of other medical conditions, particularly trauma, as observed in 20 % of cases. They are also seen in onychomycosis and even in healthy individuals with inherently delicate capillaries [4].

Leukonychia, which represents white areas of the nail due to parakeratotic foci within the nail plate, can also be a sign of psoriasis [5]. When psoriasis affects the whole matrix, the nail is distorted, rough, and friable [3, 4].

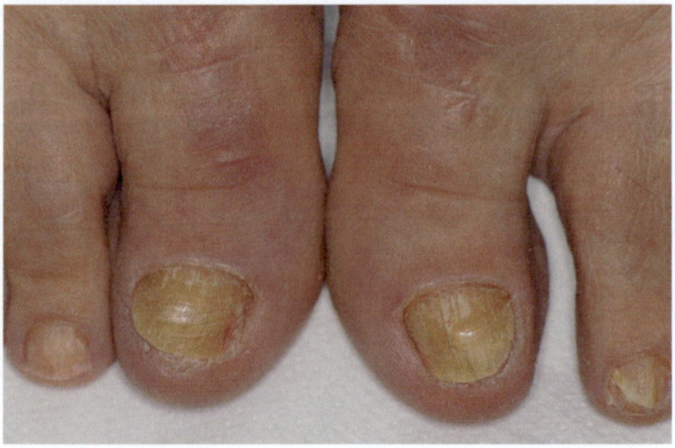

Fig. 14.3 Nail bed lichen planus. Nails are thickened and *yellow* in color; note onychorrhexis that suggests correct diagnosis

Lichen Planus

Epidemiology

Lichen planus is a chronic inflammatory disease with unknown etiology that affects the skin, hair, nails, and mucous membranes [1, 6]. The prevalence of lichen planus is not known, but is estimated to be less than 1 %. It affects women and men equally. It can occur at any age, but the majority of cases are in patients between 30 and 60 years old [7]. Lichen planus involves the nails in about 10 % of cases and can be limited to the nails only [8].

Clinical Features

Lichen planus most commonly involves the nail matrix causing longitudinal grooves and fissures, as well as progressive thinning and distal splitting of the nail plate [8]. Nail matrix destruction causes dorsal pterygium, in which the proximal nail fold adheres to the nail bed [1, 6, 9].

However, lichen planus can also affect the nail bed causing subungual hyperkeratosis and onycholysis. In the toenails it often causes yellow discoloration and thickening (yellow nail syndrome-like presentations) (Fig. 14.3). In general, patients also present signs of nail matrix involvement that suggest correct diagnosis.

Subungual Tumors

Warts

Epidemiology

Periungual warts are most commonly seen in children and teenagers, occurring most frequently in those ranging from 12 to 16 years old. There is increased incidence in those who bite their nails, who suck their fingers, and who work in a wet environment. Often, warts disappear spontaneously [10].

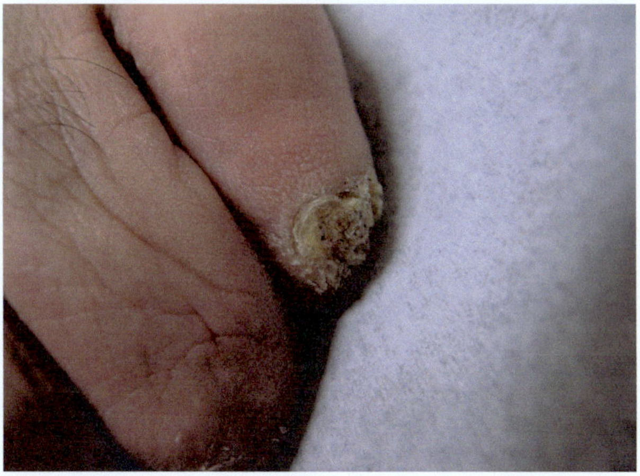

Fig. 14.4 Periungual wart

Clinical Features

Periungual warts are usually caused by HPV genotypes 1, 2, and 4. They affect fingernails more often than toenails and appear as hyperkeratotic papules with a rough surface (Fig. 14.4). Pathologically, they are characterized as having sharply demarcated hyperplasia with acanthosis, papillomatosis, and hyperkeratosis with areas of parakeratosis [10].

Initially, the warts are small in size, shiny, smooth, and translucent. Weeks to months later, they grow in size and appear rough, dirty, brownish black in color, and horny [11].

When located in the proximal nail fold, warts produce periungual hyperkeratosis forming a hyperkeratotic cuticle. Subungual warts raise the nail plate causing onycholysis and appear as a subungual nodular lesions. They may also produce a longitudinal band of onycholysis with splinter hemorrhages due to linear growth underneath the nail plate. Warts in the hyponychium of the toenails may cause distal thickening.

Warts do not affect the nail matrix, but can cause damage to it due to compression, which can cause nail plate ridging and grooving [10]. They may become fissured, inflamed, and tender and often recur after treatment [11].

Exostosis

Epidemiology

Subungual exostosis is a rare, benign osteocartilaginous tumor affecting the distal phalanx of the digits, usually the toes [12]. It presents more frequently in females and most often in the second decade of life. About one-third of patients report a history of trauma or infection at the site [13].

Clinical Features

Patients commonly present with months of pain, erythema, and onycholysis [1, 12]. It most often affects the toenails, with about 70–80 % of cases overall affecting the hallux [14].

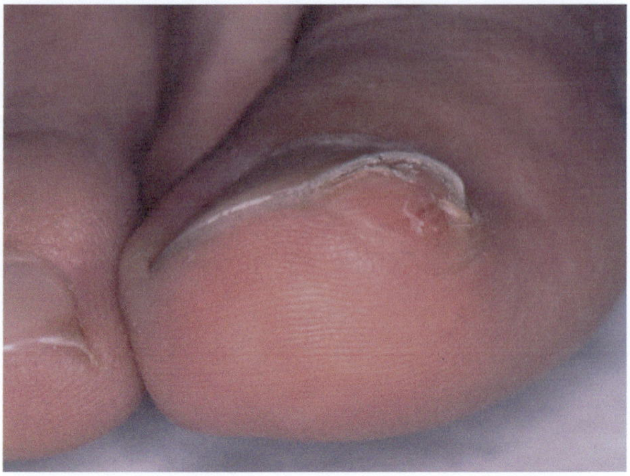

Fig. 14.5 Subungual exostosis

Examination shows a firm nodule with a hyperkeratotic and smooth surface (Fig. 14.5). The lesion is located at the distal end of the nail plate, away from the epiphyseal line. It is made of trabecular bone and is capped with fibrocartilage [12].

Squamous Cell Carcinoma

Epidemiology

Squamous cell carcinoma of the nail is rare [15]. It is most common in the fifth and sixth decades of life and tends to have a male predominance [16].

The etiology of subungual squamous cell carcinoma is unclear, although repeated trauma, chronic infection, radiation, tar, arsenic exposure, UV radiation, immunosuppression, and HPV infection may each play a role. HPV infection is particularly relevant as it is present in 60–90 % of cases [15].

Clinical Features

Subungual squamous cell carcinoma most frequently presents on the hands rather than the feet [17]. It most often involves only one digit, with the thumb and hallux being the most common [15]. The right index and middle fingers are also commonly affected [18].

Patients most commonly present with a wartlike appearance of the nail bed with nail dystrophy [15]. Nail pigmentation with longitudinal melanonychia is common (Fig. 14.6) [18].

Other clinical features include subungual hyperkeratosis, onycholysis, oozing, nail plate destruction, paronychia, leukonychia, and longitudinal erythronychia [18]. Bleeding along with nodules and ulcers may also be present [15].

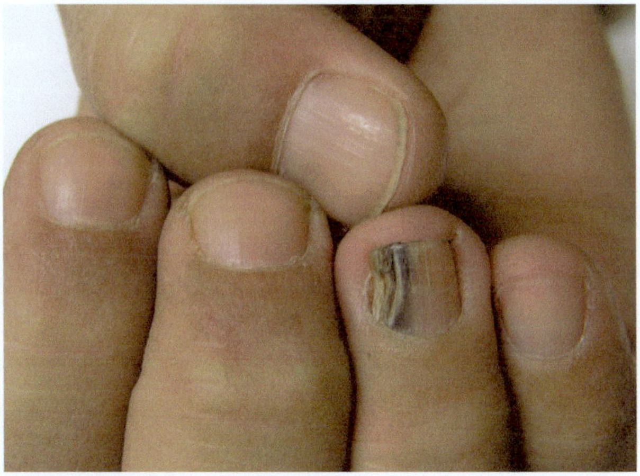

Fig. 14.6 Squamous cell carcinoma presenting with longitudinal melanonychia

Subungual Melanoma

Epidemiology

Nail melanoma is not common, as it accounts for only about 1–3 % of cutaneous melanomas diagnosed in the general population [19, 20]. Nail melanomas are seen more often in patients 50–70 years old and more often in men than women [19, 20]. Darker-skinned individuals are more commonly affected with this subtype of melanoma. Up to 75 % of cutaneous melanomas are localized in the nail in Africans, 10 % in Japanese, and 25 % in Chinese populations [20].

Clinical Features

Nail melanomas originate either from the nail matrix, or the nail bed (subungual melanomas), and may involve other parts of the nail unit such as the proximal nail fold and hyponychium. Nail matrix melanoma presents as bands of longitudinal brown-black discolorations of the nail plate (longitudinal melanonychia) [20]. The pigmented band is usually wider than 3 mm and has dishomogeneous color and blurred lateral margins (Fig. 14.7) [19, 20]. Nail bed melanoma appears as a pigmented or nonpigmented subungual nodule that initially causes nail plate detachment. It gradually enlarges, eventually leading to nail plate destruction [19]. Ulceration, pain, inflammation, discharge, and surrounding discoloration are common [20].

Hutchinson sign is a characteristic feature of invasive subungual melanoma. It is defined as extension of the dark pigment into the lateral or proximal periungual folds [1].

Nail melanomas are more often found in the hands than in the feet and most commonly in the thumb and hallux [19]. Although UV radiation is a well-known risk

Fig. 14.7 Nail matrix melanoma presenting with longitudinal melanonychia

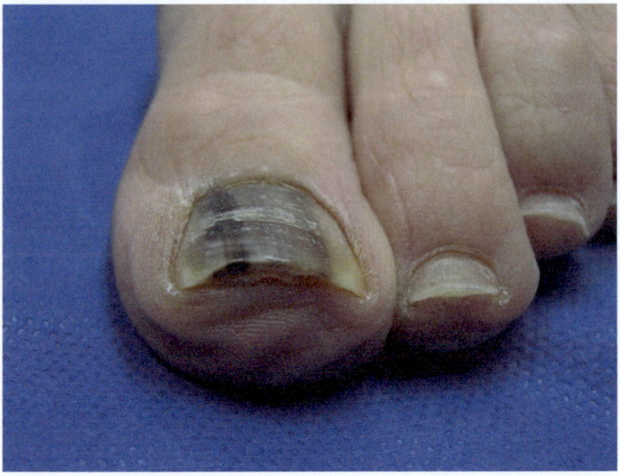

factor for cutaneous melanoma, it is unable to penetrate the nail plate and therefore is not a risk factor for subungual melanoma [19]. Instead, direct trauma to the nail is frequently reported although there is lack of evidence to form a direct correlation [20].

Contact Dermatitis

Epidemiology

Contact dermatitis can be allergic or irritant and causes inflammation of the skin due to chemical damage. It can occur at any age and is more prevalent in women and manual laborers [1].

Clinical Features

Contact dermatitis frequently affects the nail bed as chemicals penetrate through the thin onychodermal band causing subungual inflammation with onycholysis and subungual hyperkeratosis. This can be very severe in patients with contact allergy to acrylic nails (Fig. 14.8). Splinter hemorrhages are also common.

Diagnosis is suggested by the presence of periungual erythema and scaling as well as Beau's lines.

Traumatic Onycholysis

Epidemiology

Trauma of the nail unit is a common injury that can mimic onychomycosis. Trauma can be due to footwear, mechanical injury, or athletics. Traumatic nail lesions can be observed in patients of any race, sex, or age and is very commonly misdiagnosed and treated as onychomycosis.

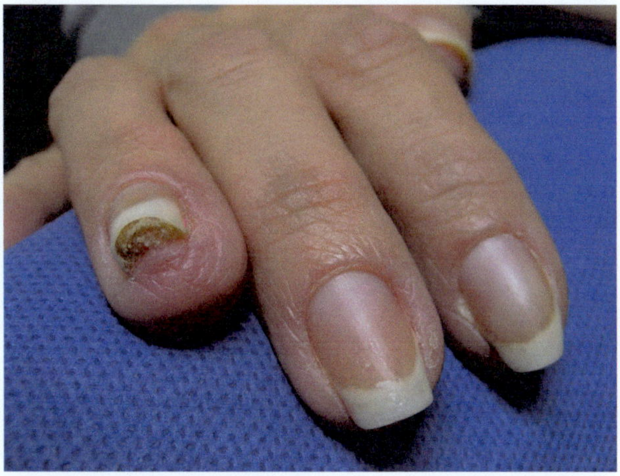

Fig. 14.8 Contact dermatitis due to acrylic nails

Clinical Features

Signs of trauma include onycholysis, subungual hyperkeratosis, abnormalities of the nail plate, changes in the hyponychium, ingrown nails, paronychia, and onychomadesis [1]. Traumatic onycholysis usually affects the big toes and is common in athletes and in women wearing high-heel shoes. It affects the lateral aspect of the toenail when caused by overlapping of the second toe or the distal nail [21] (Fig. 14.9).

It may frequently be colonized by microorganisms that produce pigments mimicking onychomycosis [2]. At dermoscopy, the proximal border of the onycholytic area is sharp.

Subungual hematoma may also occur secondary to trauma. This would produce a dark reddish-black subungual discoloration (Fig. 14.10). This discoloration would move forward and become more blue in color as the nail grows outward. Distal onycholysis and spontaneous avulsion may also occur with subungual hematoma [22]

Pachyonychia Congenita

Epidemiology

Pachyonychia congenita is a rare genetic skin disease, due to a defect in one of four keratin genes [23]. There are only an estimated 5000–10,000 cases of pachyonychia congenita reported worldwide. It affects males and females equally and has a large geographic distribution [23].

Clinical Features

Most patients with pachyonychia congenita will present with symptoms at birth or within 1 year. Three clinical features that are present in most patients regardless of mutation subtype are thickened toenails, plantar keratoderma, and plantar pain [23].

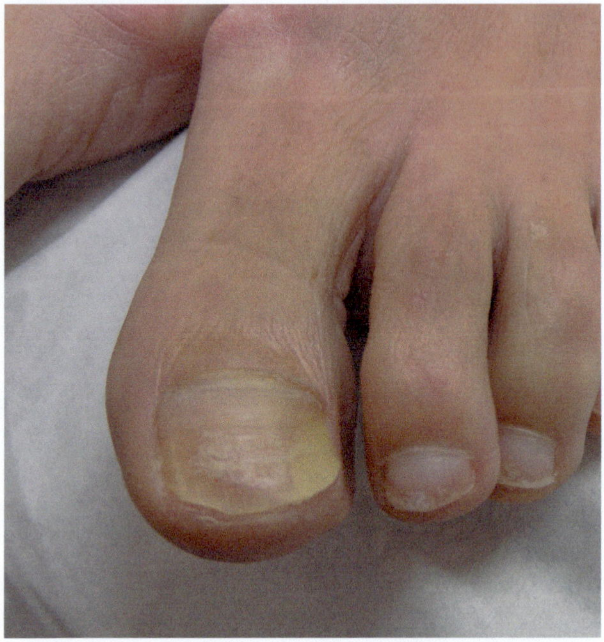

Fig. 14.9 Traumatic onycholysis due to overlapping of the second toe over the first toenail

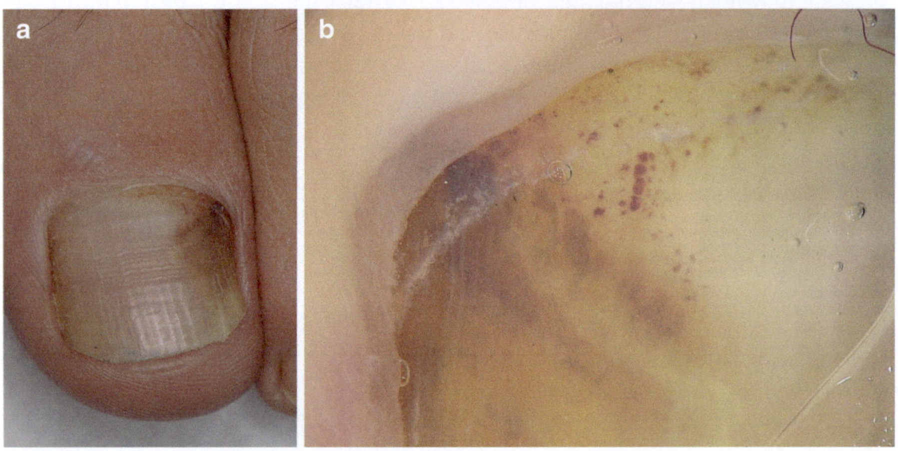

Fig. 14.10 (**a**) Traumatic onycholysis and subungual hematoma. (**b**) Dermoscopic examination showing typical red round spots due to blood extravasation

The nails show subungual hyperkeratosis in about 90–98 % of cases [1, 24]. They are very thick and develop large horns that require matrix removal in order to halt their growth [1]. Thickened toenails are the most frequently reported symptom, with the majority of the toenails being affected and in most cases all ten. Patients often file the nails to reduce the thickening (Fig. 14.11). Fingernails are less commonly affected than toenails, but may present with the same clinical features [23].

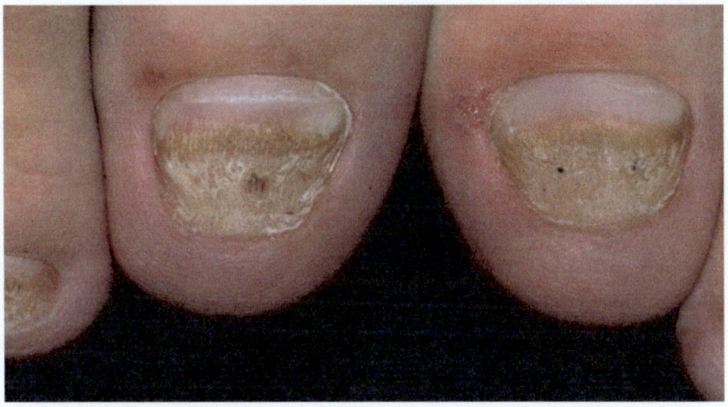

Fig. 14.11 Pachyonychia congenita affecting the toenails

Nails may also show yellowish-brown discoloration and upward angulation of the free edge of the nail plate secondary to the progressive thickening [25]. Nails may also show premature termination of the nail plate with an exposed distal fingertip [26].

Onycholysis Due to Thyroid Disease

Epidemiology

Thyroid disease is a common disorder and can be divided into two groups: hyperthyroidism and hypothyroidism. Both types can be caused by autoimmunity or iodine deficiency.

Clinical Features

Both hyperthyroidism and hypothyroidism can cause onycholysis.

Onycholysis due to hyperthyroidism is also known as Plummer's nails [27]. The hyponychium appears dirty, and brown discoloration of the nails may be seen. All of the nails of the fingers and toes are usually affected, but the fourth finger is usually the first one to show symptoms, particularly onycholysis [1].

Yellow Nail Syndrome

Epidemiology

Yellow nail syndrome is a rare disorder that presents nail abnormalities in association with lymphedema or chronic respiratory disease. Onset of yellow nail syndrome is typically seen in adulthood, most often during the fourth and sixth decade of life [28]. . Men and women are equally affected [29, 30].

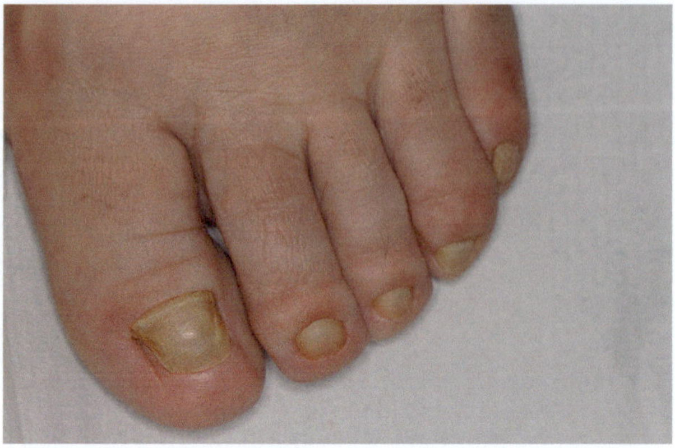

Fig. 14.12 Yellow nail syndrome

Clinical Features

Yellow nail syndrome is characterized by a triad of clinical features: yellow nails, lymphedema, and chronic respiratory involvement (pleural effusion, bronchiectasis, sinus infection, chronic cough, and chronic lung infections). Two of these features must be present in order to make a diagnosis of yellow nail syndrome [1, 28].

Nails are primarily affected with yellow discoloration and arrested or abnormally slow growth. The cuticle is absent and the nails are overcurved, and onycholysis is common (Fig. 14.12) [31]. The nail changes are reversible and might resolve spontaneously, with control of the respiratory symptoms or of the lymphedema [29, 30].

Drug-Induced Onycholysis

Epidemiology

Cutaneous drug reactions account for 10–30 % of all adverse drug reactions. Women and men are affected equally, and the possibility of cutaneous adverse drug reactions tends to increase with age [32].

The most popular drugs causing nail abnormalities include tetracyclines, psoralens, quinolones, and taxanes [33].

Clinical Features

Drug-induced nail changes usually affect most or all of the nails, on both the hands and feet. Nail changes are frequently reversible upon drug withdrawal, except discoloration which can remain for years.

Tetracyclines rarely cause photo-onycholysis, which occurs after drug ingestion and exposure to UV light. Photo-onycholysis causes nail plate detachment with

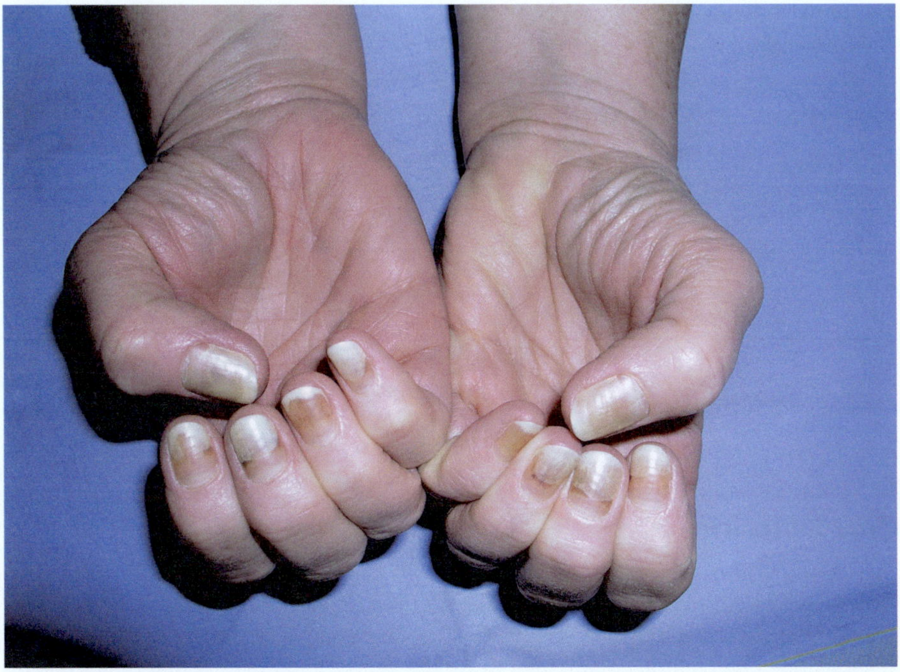

Fig. 14.13 Hemorrhagic onycholysis due to taxanes

subungual hemorrhages. It most often affects the fingernails meanwhile sparing the thumb and will involve the toenails if they are exposed to the sun. Pain may be present in some patients, as well as a convex-shaped nail. It usually appears after 2 or 3 weeks of taking the drug, and symptoms may occur even after discontinuation of the drug. Other drugs that are known to cause photo-onycholysis are psoralens, quinolones, chloramphenicol, and NSAIDs [1, 34].

Onycholysis can result from damage to the nail bed or formation of hemorrhagic bulla due to drug reactions. The hemorrhagic bulla can be painful, but fortunately the nail resolves upon drug withdrawal. Drugs that can cause this condition include psoralens, retinoids, and chemotherapeutic drugs [33].

Taxanes commonly cause painful hemorrhagic onycholysis with subungual exudation (Fig. 14.13).

Proximal Subungual Onychomycosis

The differential diagnosis includes diseases that cause true leukonychia and proximal onycholysis.

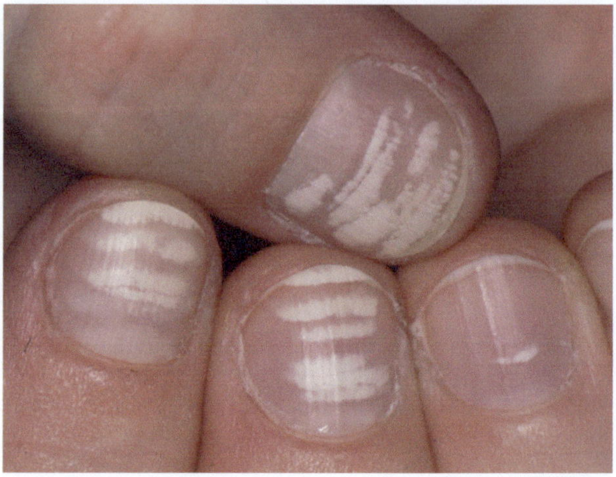

Fig. 14.14 Transverse leukonychia due to manicure

True Leukonychia

True leukonychia is caused by abnormal nail plate maturation with the presence of parakeratotic cells within the nail plate. Traumas and hereditary conditions can be responsible. Overzealous manicures cause transverse leukonychia that might resemble recurrent bands of proximal subungual onychomycosis (Fig. 14.14).

Proximal Onycholysis

This can be a consequence of trauma. The proximal nail is white because of the presence of air, but the color is not opaque white as it is in leukonychia from proximal subungual onychomycosis.

White Subungual Onychomycosis

Pseudo-leukonychia

Brittle nails due to continuous wearing of nail polish may present with white patches of pseudo-leukonychia due to superficial keratin degranulation that looks similar to white superficial onychomycosis (Fig. 14.15). However, keratin degranulation is usually seen in fingernails, and it is important to keep in mind that this type of onychomycosis is exclusively seen in toenails.

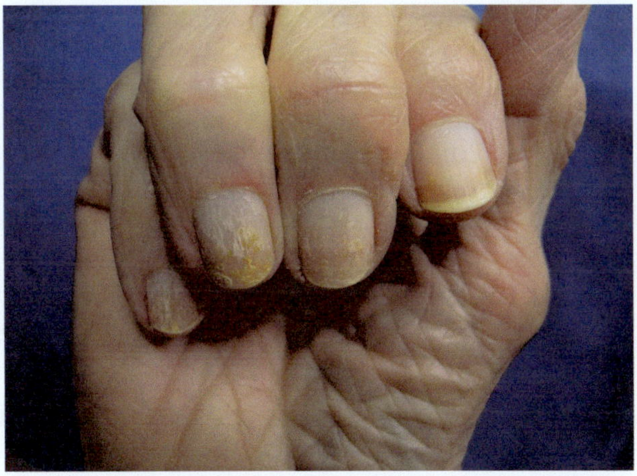

Fig. 14.15 Pseudo-leukonychia due to repeated use of nail polish

Diagnostic Clues

In general, onychomycosis is unlikely when all toenails are affected, fingernails of both hands are affected, and subungual nodules are present.

Psoriasis: look for pitting/salmon patches, skin/scalp involvement, and joint enlargement/pain.

Nail bed lichen planus: look for signs of nail matrix involvement.

Nail melanoma: utilize ABCDEF guidelines and brown/black color with irregular lines at dermoscopy (Table 14.1).

Contact dermatitis: usually fingernails, periungual skin frequently affected.

Table 14.1 ABCDEF guidelines for diagnosis of subungual melanoma

A	*A*ge: peaks at 50–70 years old Race: *A*frican-*A*merican, Native *A*merican, *A*sian
B	*B*and *B*rown-*b*lack pigment *B*readth of band > 3 mm *B*order is irregular/blurred
C	*C*hange: in size and growth rate Lack of *c*hange: failure of nail dystrophy to improve with treatment
D	*D*ominant hand *D*igit involved: thumb > hallux > index finger Single digit > multiple digits affected
E	*E*xtension of pigment discoloration (Hutchinson sign)
F	*F*amily (or personal) history of melanoma

Traumatic onycholysis: look for podiatric abnormalities including hallux valgus/ overlapping of second toe on first toe (Greek foot)/round dark spots corresponding to hematoma at dermoscopy.

Pachyonychia congenita: onset during early infancy, nail thickening without onycholysis, and severe pain.

Onycholysis in thyroid disease: several fingernails commonly affected.

Yellow nail syndrome: arrested nail growth, most fingernails usually affected.

Drug-induced onycholysis: all nails usually involved, often hemorrhagic.

True leukonychia: many nails involved, cuticle damaged when caused by traumas.

Pseudo-leukonychia: usually fingernails (not affected by WSO), staining from nail polish commonly associated.

Summary for the Clinician

Fungal infection leads to onychodystrophic nails only about 50 % of the time [1]. The other 50 % of onychodystrophic nails may be attributed to the clinical mimickers of onychomycosis, all outlined above. It is important for the clinician to be aware of these mimickers when diagnosing the patient and selecting treatments, as the various conditions require different treatments.

Onychodystrophies can have significant effects on patients' emotional, social, and occupational behaviors because of their esthetic effects or pain [2]. Therefore, misdiagnosis can prolong these effects, and the infection may worsen, representing the need for correct diagnosis in a timely manner.

Clinical Pearls

It is not onychomycosis when:

- All nails are involved.
- All fingernails are involved.
- Onycholysis is not associated with subungual hyperkeratosis.
- Proximal border of onycholysis is sharp.

References

1. Allevato MA. Diseases mimicking onychomycosis. Clin Dermatol. 2010;28(2):164–77. doi:10.1016/j.clindermatol.2009.12.001. Review
2. Elewski BE. Onychomycosis: pathogenesis, diagnosis, and management. Clin Microbiol Rev. 1998;11(3):415–29.
3. Bloom R, Tosti A. The clinical features of nail psoriasis. In: Rigopoulus D, Tosti A, editors. Nail psoriasis from A to Z. Cham: Springer Verlag Heidelberg; 2014. p. 43–56.
4. Jiaravuthisan MM, Sasseville D, Vender RB, Murphy F, Muhn CY. Psoriasis of the nail: anatomy, pathology, clinical presentation, and a review of the literature on therapy. J Am Acad Dermatol. 2007;57(1):1–27. Review

5. Li C. Epidemiology of nail psoriasis. In: Nail psoriasis. Medscape. 2015. http://emedicine.medscape.com/article/1107949-overview#a3. Accessed 25 Mar 2016.
6. Gorouhi F, Davari P, Fazel N. Cutaneous and mucosal lichen planus: a comprehensive review of clinical subtypes, risk factors, diagnosis, and prognosis. Scientific World Journal. 2014;1–22 doi:10.1155/2014/742826.
7. Wagner G, Rose C, Sachse MM. Clinical variants of lichen planus. J Dtsch Dermatol Ges. 2013;11(4):309–19. doi:10.1111/ddg.12031. Epub 2013 Jan 15. Review
8. Tosti A, Peluso AM, Fanti PA, Piraccini BM. Nail lichen planus: clinical and pathologic study of twenty-four patients. J Am Acad Dermatol. 1993;28(5 Pt 1):724–30.
9. Tosti A, Daniel R, Piraccini BM, Iorizzo M. Nail lichen planus. In: Color Atlas of nails. Berlin: Springer; 2010. p. 83.
10. Tosti A, Piraccini BM. Warts of the nail unit: surgical and nonsurgical approaches. Dermatol Surg. 2001;27(3):235–9. Review
11. Patidar S. Combination treatment of periungual warts. J Cutan Aesthet Surg. 2008;1(1):23–4. doi:10.4103/0974-2077.41154.
12. DaCambra MP, Gupta SK, Ferri-de-Barros F. A novel management strategy for subungual exostosis. BMJ Case Rep. 2013;2013:bcr2013200396. doi:10.1136/bcr-2013-200396.
13. Olvi LG, Gonzalez ML, Santini-Araujo E. Subungual exostosis. Tumors and tumor-Like lesions of bone. London: Springer; 2015. p. 847.
14. Ward CM, Dittmer A. Subungual exotosis of the finger: case report and review of the literature. Iowa Orthop J. 2013;33:228–31.
15. Batalla A, Feal C, Rosón E, Posada C. Subungual squamous cell carcinoma: a case series. Indian J Dermatol. 2014;59(4):352–4. doi:10.4103/0019-5154.135480.
16. Abner S, Redstone J, Chowdhry S, Kasdan ML, Wilhelmi BJ. Synchronous squamous cell carcinoma in multiple digits. Eplasty. 2011;11:e9.
17. Attiyeh FF, Shah J, Booher RJ, Knapper WH. Subungual squamous cell carcinoma. JAMA. 1979;241(3):262–3.
18. Lecerf P, Richert B, Theunis A, André J. A retrospective study of squamous cell carcinoma of the nail unit diagnosed in a Belgian general hospital over a 15-year period. J Am Acad Dermatol. 2013;69(2):253–61. doi:10.1016/j.jaad.2013.02.008. Epub 2013 Apr 9
19. Tang CYK, Fung BKK, Lung CP. A hidden threat: subungual melanoma in hand. Surg Sci. 2012;3(2):78–83.
20. Patel GA, Ragi G, Krysicki J, Schwartz RA. Subungual melanoma: a deceptive disorder. Acta Dermatovenerol Croat. 2008;16(4):236–42. Review
21. Zaias N, Escovar SX, Zaiac MN. Finger and toenail onycholysis. J Eur Acad Dermatol Venereol. 2015;29(5):848–53. Daniel CR 3rd, Iorizzo M, Piraccini BM, Tosti A. Simple onycholysis. Cutis. 2011;87(5):226–8.
22. Abdullah L, Abbas O. Common nail changes and disorders in older people: diagnosis and management. Can Fam Physician. 2011;57(2):173–81.
23. Eliason MJ, Leachman SA, Feng BJ, Schwartz ME, Hansen CD. A review of the clinical phenotype of 254 patients with genetically confirmed pachyonychia congenita. J Am Acad Dermatol. 2012;67(4):680–6. doi:10.1016/j.jaad.2011.12.009. Epub 2012 Jan 20
24. Agarwal P, Chhaperwal MK, Singh A, et al. Pachyonychia congenita: a rare genodermatosis. Indian Dermatol Online J. 2013;4(3):225–7. doi:10.4103/2229-5178.115527.
25. Inamadar AC, Palit A. Nails: diagnostic clue to genodermatoses. Indian J Dermatol Venereol Leprol. 2012;78:271–8.
26. Smith FJD, Hansen CD, Hull PR, et al. Pachyonychia congenita. 2006 Jan 27 [Updated 2014 Jul 24]. In: Pagon RA, Adam MP, Ardinger HH, et al., editors. GeneReviews® [Internet]. Seattle (WA): University of Washington, Seattle; 1993–2016. Available from: http://www.ncbi.nlm.nih.gov/books/NBK1280/?report=classic.
27. Safer JD. Thyroid hormone action on skin. Dermatoendocrinol. 2011;3(3):211–5. doi:10.4161/derm.3.3.17027.
28. Chavda LK, Vaidya RA, Vaidya AD. Yellow nail syndrome: missed diagnosis of a rare syndrome. J Assoc Physicians India. 2011;59:258–60.

29. Maldonado F, Tazelaar HD, Wang CW, Ryu JH. Yellow nail syndrome: analysis of 41 consecutive patients. Chest. 2008;134(2):375–81. doi:10.1378/chest.08-0137.
30. Maldonado F, Ryu JH. Yellow nail syndrome. Curr Opin Pulm Med. 2009;15(4):371–5. doi:10.1097/MCP.0b013e32832ad45a. Review
31. Hershko A, Hirshberg B, Nahir M, Friedman G. Yellow nail syndrome. Postgrad Med J. 1997;73(862):466–8. Review
32. Choon SE, Lai NM. An epidemiological and clinical analysis of cutaneous adverse drug reactions seen in a tertiary hospital in Johor, Malaysia. Indian J Dermatol Venereol Leprol. 2012;78:734–9.
33. Piraccini BM, Tosti A. Drug-induced nail disorders: incidence, management and prognosis. Drug Saf. 1999;21(3):187–201. Review
34. Al-Kathiri L, Al-Asmaili A. Diclofenac-induced photo-onycholysis. Oman Med J. 2016;31(1):65–8. doi:10.5001/omj.2016.12.

Part III
How to Provide Best Treatment

Chapter 15
Prognostic Factors

Chris G. Adigun and Tracey C. Vlahovic

Onychomycosis treatment is challenging, as many patients do not respond to therapeutic intervention, and of those that do respond, recurrence of disease occurs frequently. There are a number of factors that contribute to these therapeutic failures. Understanding these factors is key for effective patient education on their treatment options, setting their expectations for likelihood of response, and for developing strategies to prevent recurrence at the conclusion of therapy.

There are multiple prognostic factors that play a central role in determining how effectively a patient will respond to the treatment. A key factor is the severity of the nail disease. Determining the severity of onychomycosis disease is a critical part of the evaluation and ability to predict response to treatment. A patient with only mild disease is more likely to respond to treatment than a patient with moderate disease; and similarly, a patient with moderate disease has a better chance of responding to treatment than does a patient with severe disease [1]. Major features that contribute to onychomycosis disease severity include percentage of nail involvement, matrix involvement, existence of a dermatophytoma, and degree of subungual hyperkeratosis. These are the parameters that contribute to the onychomycosis severity index (OSI) [1]. An additional factor of the nail disease that contributes to prognosis is the number of nails involved. The more nails involved, the more extensive is the disease and the poorer is the prognosis. Long-standing infections tend to be more severe, as spontaneous resolution of onychomycosis is rare and disease duration is often >5 years [2].

However, there are a number of factors that contribute to a patient's onychomycosis prognosis that are independent of the severity of their nail disease. These include patient behaviors such as risk for nail trauma from shoe selection, participation in

C.G. Adigun, MD
Board Certified Dermatologist and Nail Specialist, Chapel Hill, NC, USA

T.C. Vlahovic, DPM, FFPM RCPS (Glasg) (✉)
Department of Podiatric Medicine, Temple University School of Podiatric Medicine, Philadelphia, PA, USA
e-mail: traceyv@temple.edu

A. Tosti et al. (eds.), *Onychomycosis*, DOI 10.1007/978-3-319-44853-4_15

sports, and hygiene behaviors [2, 3]. Nail trauma facilitates invasion of the dermatophyte by providing an uninhibited pathway of infection. Chronic nail trauma, or a chronically malformed nail, potentially is forever vulnerable to infection, making sustained clearance incredibly difficult [4].

In addition, factors related to the patient's health status are critical to the prognostic evaluation. Comorbid conditions such as old age [5], diabetes mellitus [6, 7], peripheral vascular disease [8, 9], and/or psoriasis [2] all portend a poor response to treatment. These conditions often lead to slow or poor nail growth, due to poor circulation, and/or chronic nail trauma, due to diabetic neuropathy or arthritic gate abnormalities.

Immunosuppression, whether due to a complication from diabetes mellitus, autoimmune disease, HIV, or iatrogenic, contributes to poor response to treatment for onychomycosis [10, 11]. Patients that are immunosuppressed due to one or more of these factors need to be prepared for the possibility of treatment failure.

A genetic predisposition to superficial fungal infections has been established [12, 13]. The evidence that onychomycosis has a genetic component originates from the observation that among individuals exposed to identical environmental conditions and fungal pathogens, some do not develop onychomycosis, whereas others go on to develop chronic infections [12, 14]. The genetic component that contributes to this susceptibility to chronic disease is thought to be located in the innate or adaptive immune system. Defects in the innate or adaptive immune response to dermatophytes prevent the subsequent development of the full immune response, thereby rendering the individual vulnerable to this infection [13].

There are a number of genetic mutations that have been identified that increase an individual's susceptibility to superficial dermatophyte infection, including onychomycosis. These include mutations in the innate immune receptors dectin-1 and its adaptor protein CARD9 [13]. There are specific human leukocyte antigen (HLA) genotypes that have been identified as more common in families with higher prevalence of onychomycosis. In addition, patients with insufficient levels of CD4+CD25+ regulatory T cells have an impaired immune response to superficial dermatophyte infection [13].

Our understanding of the factors that contribute to more persistent cases onychomycosis continues to evolve. At the same time, the landscape of therapeutic options for this multifactorial disease is in congruent evolution as we learn optimal ways of treating and managing this disease. There are a number of factors that portend a poor prognosis for those afflicted with onychomycosis. In addition to the severity of the infection, the largest players include old age, diabetes mellitus, peripheral vascular disease, immunosuppression, nail trauma, and genetic predisposition. Patient education is paramount in managing expectations to treatment response. It is important for both providers and patients to recognize that treatment failure is more likely to be due to one or more of these varieties of host factors rather than the susceptibility of their infective organism to the antifungal treatment.

References

1. Carney C, Tosti A, Daniel R, Scher R, Rich P, DeCoster J, Elewski B. A new classification system for grading the severity of onychomycosis: Onychomycosis Severity Index. Arch Dermatol. 2011;147(11):1277–82.
2. Rosen T, Friedlander SF, Kircik L, Zirwas MJ, Stein Gold L, Bhatia N, Gupta AK. Onychomycosis: epidemiology, diagnosis, and treatment in a changing landscape. J Drugs Dermatol. 2015;14(3):223–33.
3. Gupta AK, Lynch LE. Onychomycosis: review of recurrence rates, poor prognostic factors, and strategies to prevent disease recurrence. Cutis. 2004;74(1 Suppl):10–5.
4. Svejgaard EL, Nilsson J. Onychomycosis in Denmark: prevalence of fungal nail infection in general practice. Mycoses. 2004;47(3-4):131–5.
5. Loo DS. Onychomycosis in the elderly : drug treatment options. Drugs Aging. 2007;24(4): 293–302.
6. Mayser P, Freund V, Budihardja D. Toenail onychomycosis in diabetic patients: issues and management. Am J Clin Dermatol. 2009;10(4):211–20.
7. Papini M, Cicoletti M, Fabrizi V, Landucci P. Skin and nail mycoses in patients with diabetic foot. G Ital Dermatol Venereol. 2013;148(6):603–8.
8. Ozkan F, Ozturk P, Ozyurt K, İncı MF, Kalender AM, Bakan B, Yuksel M. Frequency of peripheral arterial disease and venous insufficiency in toenail onychomycosis. J Dermatol. 2013;40(2):107–10.
9. Gupta AK, Gupta MA, Summerbell RC, Cooper EA, Konnikov N, Albreski D, MacDonald P, Harris KA. The epidemiology of onychomycosis: possible role of smoking and peripheral arterial disease. J Eur Acad Dermatol Venereol. 2000;14(6):466–9.
10. Cribier BJ, Bakshi R. Terbinafine in the treatment of onychomycosis: a review of its efficacy in high-risk populations and in patients with nondermatophyte infections. Br J Dermatol. 2004;150(3):414–20.
11. Tuchinda P, Boonchai W, Prukpaisarn P, Maungprasat C, Suthipinittharm P. Prevalence of onychomycosis in patients with autoimmune diseases. J Med Assoc Thail. 2006;89(8): 1249–52.
12. Faergemann J, Correia O, Nowicki R, Ro BI. Genetic predisposition – understanding underlying mechanisms of onychomycosis. J Eur Acad Dermatol Venereol. 2005;19(Suppl 1):17–9.
13. Gupta AK, Simpson FC, Brintnell WC. Do genetic mutations and genotypes contribute to onychomycosis? Dermatology. 2014;228(3):207–10.
14. Zaias N, Tosti A, Rebell G, Morelli R, Bardazzi F, Bieley H, Zaiac M, Glick B, Paley B, Allevato M, Baran R. Autosomal dominant pattern of distal subungual onychomycosis caused by Trichophyton rubrum. J Am Acad Dermatol. 1996;34(2 Pt 1):302–4.

Chapter 16
Why Onychomycosis Can Be a Life-Threatening Condition

Tracey C. Vlahovic, Christina Bui, and Kyle Shaw

Onychomycosis is often mistaken by both physicians and patients as being not only a cosmetic entity but also of secondary or tertiary importance in the patient's list of concerns. This book has strived to show that it is an infection which affects a wide range of patients. It may not present itself as a carbuncle or a circumscribed area of cellulitis, but its simple presence can indicate something more sinister such as the link to carotid atherosclerosis in diabetics or create an environment where a dermatophyte can infect the interdigital space leading to a possible bacterial superinfection [1, 2].

Cellulitis, commonly seen on the lower extremity in older adults with diabetes, is a diagnosis that requires a hospital admission in cases that are potentially limb and life threatening [3]. The link to lower extremity cellulitis from a mycotic toenail may not seem logical at first, but in some cases, that fungal foot infection provided the initial spark for a problematic chain reaction.

The presence of onychomycosis generally co-presents with tinea pedis, specifically interdigital tinea pedis. It can be difficult to know which caused the other, but a general statement can be made that the same dermatophyte, whether starting from the nail or the interdigital space, is creating both the infection in the nail bed and the plantar/toe-web skin. When examining a patient with onychomycosis, it is worthwhile for the practitioner to examine the skin around the nail, interdigital space, and plantar foot for the serpiginous scale characteristic of tinea pedis. The patient may not have symptoms of pruritus, but in some cases, the skin will not only present with the characteristic scale but may also present with mild inflammation and fissuring [3]. The fissures can act as a portal for bacteria to invade and create an infectious and inflammatory cascade.

T.C. Vlahovic, DPM, FFPM RCPS (Glasg) (✉)
Department of Podiatric Medicine, Temple University School of Podiatric Medicine, 148 N 8th Street, Philadelphia, 19107 PA, USA
e-mail: traceyv@temple.edu

C. Bui, BA • K. Shaw, BS
Department of Podiatric Medicine, Temple University School of Podiatric Medicine, Philadelphia, PA, USA
e-mail: Christina.bui@temple.edu; tuf22898@temple.edu

A. Tosti et al. (eds.), *Onychomycosis*, DOI 10.1007/978-3-319-44853-4_16

Bristow and Spruce reviewed the literature to determine the potentiality of a fungal foot infection causing cellulitis, especially in the diabetic population [3]. One of the articles they reviewed was Roujeau et al.'s case-controlled study of 243 patients with acute bacterial cellulitis of the leg that aimed to find any association with mycology-proven foot dermatomycosis (i.e., both tinea pedis and onychomycosis) [4]. The presence of a fungal foot infection was a significant risk factor in developing cellulitis with an odds ratio of 2.4, $p < 0.001$, confidence interval 95 % [4]. Another prospective case-controlled study of 100 subjects concluded that risk factors for acute bacterial cellulitis in hospitalized patients were sites of pathogen entry on legs and toe webs. Therefore, management and treatment of toe-web intertrigo may reduce cellulitis incidence [5]. Likewise, Dupuy et al. assessed risk factors for erysipelas of the leg, cellulitis, through seven hospital centers in France [6]. One hundred and sixty seven patients were admitted for erysipelas of the leg, and through multivariate analysis, they showed that disruption of the cutaneous barrier secondary to a macerated interdigital space was a risk factor in developing cellulitis (odds ratio 6.6, 95 % confidence interval). A site of entry through the skin was found in almost all cases. In the same study, the risk of developing leg cellulitis increased when more than one interdigital space was affected (odds ratio 19.5, 95 % confidence interval).

Ultimately, Bristow and Spruce found 16 studies that supported the presence of a fungal foot infection as a risk factor for cellulitis. This included examining patients with toe-web tinea pedis, onychomycosis, and plantar tinea pedis (moccasin type). More specifically, the association of interdigital tinea pedis was consistently a predictive factor in developing cellulitis; however, the more sites fungally infected increased the risk even more as in Dupuy et al.'s article. Some of the studies, most of them involving hospital patients, grouped nail disease with the general term "fungal foot infection." Population-attributable risk (PAR) of bacterial cellulitis was highest for toe-web intertrigo at 60 %. The PAR is the percentage of cases of bacterial cellulitis that could possibly be avoided if the risk factor was removed. Tinea pedis and concomitant mycological infection of the nail, onychomycosis, are the components of the highly prevalent condition of toe-web intertrigo.

Therefore, even though interdigital tinea pedis is associated with a slightly higher risk to develop cellulitis than plantar tinea pedis or onychomycosis alone, the presence of onychomycosis whether currently or in that patient's future can't be ruled out. These are skin manifestations that present together and must be joined in the practitioner's mind.

In addition to the toe-web spaces acting as a portal of entry for bacteria, an ulceration from the pressure of the thickened, mycotic nail in shoe gear must also be considered. Sharp edges of onychauxic toenails that are often unnoticed in a neuropathic diabetic patient can create ulcerations and abrasions that may become superinfected with bacteria, a perfect storm created by lack of sensation and the humid nature of wearing shoes colonized with various flora for most of the day. The jagged or sharp edges of the nail plate that are abutting onto the surrounding digits could lead to an ulceration [7]. Depending on the vascular status of the patient, this ulceration may become gangrenous and may develop osteomyelitis or cellulitis which in theory could lead to a possible amputation of not just the digit but also the limb. In addition to the surrounding digits being affected, the nail bed of the mycotic toenail may break down with repeated trauma and pressure. Again, this ulceration may prove to be a limb-threatening situation if it becomes infected or if the patient's health and vascular status do not support a healthy healing environment. A potential patient population to illustrate this scenario is the diabetic. Chadwick et al. made a link between diabetes and the development of a fungal infection contributing to the pathogenesis of ulceration and cellulitis in a diabetic foot [8]. He encourages that fungal foot infections in a diabetic should not be ignored or considered cosmetic, and as consistent in the literature, they have a high risk of secondary bacterial infection. Also, the consequences of fungal foot infections for those with peripheral neurological and/or vascular status are exacerbated in addition to their diabetic condition and sequela. Therefore, treatment for the fungal infection should be initiated immediately, and preventative measures (such as managing environment, socks, and shoes) should be discussed.

Lastly, Doyle et al. state that there is a higher incidence of foot ulceration and gangrene in diabetic patients with onychomycosis versus those who do not [9]. These scenarios support the periodic physician-based examination of the lower extremity as well as the diabetic patient's daily inspection of their feet (and socks) for any drainage, cuts, tears, or redness.

Overall, the presence of onychomycosis, which can lead to interdigital tinea pedis that morphs into a bacterially superinfected toe web, may create a potentially limb and life-threatening situation, especially in the diabetic population. Onychomycosis itself is a visually displeasing entity but, for a certain subset of patients, may prove to be something much more problematic. It is an infection and should be treated with the same care and respect that similar maladies are managed.

References

1. Onalan O, Adar A, Keles H, Ertugrul G, Ozkan N, Aktas H, Karakaya E. Onychomycosis is associated with subclinical atherosclerosis in patients with diabetes. Vasa. 2015;44(1): 59–64.
2. Tan JS, Joseph WS. Common fungal infections of the feet in patients with diabetes mellitus. Drugs Aging. 2004;21(2):101–12.
3. Bristow IR, Spruce MC. Fungal Foot Infection, cellulitis, and diabetes: a review. Diabet Med. 2009;26:548–51.
4. Roujeau JC, Sigurgeirsson B, Korting HC, Kerl H, Paul C. Chronic dermatomycoses of the foot as risk factors for acute bacterial cellulitis of the leg: a case-control study. Dermatology. 2004;209(4):301–7.
5. Björnsdóttir S, Gottfredsson M, Thórisdóttir AS, Gunnarsson GB, Ríkardsdóttir H, Kristjánsson M, Hilmarsdóttir I. Risk factors for acute cellulitis of the lower limb: a prospective case-control study. Clin Infect Dis. 2005;41(10):1416–22.

6. Dupuy A, Benchikhi H, Roujeau J-C, Bernard P, Vaillant L, Chosidow O, Sassolas BR, Guillaume J-C, Grob J-J, Bastuni-Garin S. Risk factors for erysipelas of the leg (cellulitis): case-control study. BMJ. 1999;318:1591–4.
7. Gulcan A, Gulcan E, Oksuz S, Sahin I, Kaya D. Prevalence of toenail onychomycosis in patients with type 2 diabetes mellitus and evaluation of risk factors. JAPMA. 2011;101(1):49.
8. Chadwick P. Fungal infection of the diabetic foot: the often ignored complication. Diabet Foot Can. 2013;1(2):20–4.
9. Doyle JJ, Boyko WL, Ryu S et al. Onychomycosis among diabetic patients: prevalence and impact of nonfungal foot infections. ADA 6th annual scientific session; 9–13 Jun 2000; San Antonio. ADA, 2000.

Chapter 17
Onychomycosis in Diabetics

Tracey C. Vlahovic and Joshua A. Sebag

Epidemiology and Risk Factors

According to the American Diabetes Association, there are approximately 29.1 million Americans or 9.3 % of the population that suffer from diabetes [1]. Twenty-one million have already been diagnosed with the disease, and 8.1 million remain undiagnosed [1]. This number pales in comparison to the 86 million Americans who have been classified as "prediabetic," i.e., those who are on the borderline of becoming diabetic in the future. Within this subset of patients, pedal complaints, such as painful, thickened toenails are of chief concern as onychomycosis is much more than a cosmetic issue. In the diabetic population, the diagnosis and management of the fungal toenail may be overlooked as more medically pertinent findings like concomitant renal disease, cardiovascular risk factors, retinopathy, and diabetic foot wounds usurp the practitioner's time. However, if onychomycosis is overlooked and not properly managed in these patients, it can become a limb-threatening condition [2].

In the general population, estimations of mycotic toenail infections vary, but one epidemiologic survey reported an overall disease prevalence of 2–13 % with evidence of a steadily rising incidence worldwide [3]. The prevalence of diabetic vs nondiabetic patients with onychomycosis was shown to be statistically significant at 17 and 6.8 %, respectively. Almost a threefold increase was appreciated in those patients that had diabetes mellitus when it came to having clinically evident toenail fungus [4]. Looking at prevalence and risk factors, onychomycosis was present in

T.C. Vlahovic, DPM, FFPM RCPS (Glasg) (✉)
Department of Podiatric Medicine, Temple University School of Podiatric Medicine,
148 N 8th Street, Philadelphia, 19107 PA, USA
e-mail: traceyv@temple.edu

J.A. Sebag, BA
Department of Podiatric Medicine, Temple University School
of Podiatric Medicine, Philadelphia, PA, USA
e-mail: Sebag.Josh@gmail.com

A. Tosti et al. (eds.), *Onychomycosis*, DOI 10.1007/978-3-319-44853-4_17

26 % of diabetics of the time [5]. Further projections were made, and approximately one-third of the overall subjects with a diagnosis of diabetes were affected [5].

General predisposing factors in developing onychomycosis include increasing age, male gender, family history of onychomycosis, concurrent intake of immunosuppressive agents, and peripheral vascular disease [6]. Onychomycosis is the most common skin issue in a diabetic patient [6]. Also, in this population, mycotic nails are often associated with hyperlipidemia, peripheral artery disease, diabetes duration, metabolic syndrome, obesity, smoking, and atherosclerosis [7]. Onalan et al. examined 127 patients with diabetes type 2 [7]. Of those patients, 48 had onychomycosis (37.8 %), and 60 had subclinical atherosclerosis of the carotid (47.2 %). After further investigation, they concluded that "the presence of toenail onychomycosis is independently associated with the presence of subclinical atherosclerosis" as seen in the carotid intima-media thickness in patients with diabetes [7]. Therefore, toenail disease in diabetics can be a marker of something much more sinister but ultimately screenable and, in theory, treatable if caught early.

In addition to it being a marker for atherosclerosis, mycotic toenails may also pose a problem when the patient is neuropathic. Long-standing hyperglycemia affects cellular immunity, which may predispose a diabetic to fungal invasion [8]. Increasing nail thickness is associated with a higher hemoglobin A1C (HgA1C) value [9]. One of the most frequent diabetic complications is a diabetic foot ulcer, especially in a neurovascular compromised patient. A sharp-edged, thickened toenail that would be perceived as such in a sensate patient could go unnoticed in a neuropathic diabetic patient. This could lead to an ulceration of the nail bed or erosions of the surrounding tissue or digits that are exposed to the jagged or sharp edges of the nail plate [8]. Depending on the vascular status of the patient, this ulceration may become gangrenous and may develop osteomyelitis or cellulitis which in theory could lead to a possible amputation of not just the digit but also the limb. Doyle et al. state that there is a higher incidence of foot ulceration and gangrene in diabetic patients with onychomycosis versus those who do not [10]. This justifies the need for proper and routine foot screenings and care, as simply debriding the nails and inspecting the pedal skin on a regular basis could be limb saving in certain cases.

Unique to the lower extremity, studies have suggested that confining shoe gear and systemic immunosuppression increase the susceptibility of onychomycosis with varying levels of morbidity in the diabetic foot [11–13]. In the confines of the shoe, faulty foot and ankle biomechanics add another risk to developing nail disease. Onychomycosis is most commonly found in the hallux toenail in comparison to the lesser toenails [14]. Normal pedal ambulation and biomechanics rely on the hallux acting in the propulsive cycle as a rigid lever arm [13]. If the first metatarsophalangeal joint is limited in either a dorsiflexory or plantarflexory direction, the hallux nail can become compromised due to chronic repetitive trauma which may lead to fungal invasion [15]. In the case of a diabetic with neuropathy, the pain that this joint limitation would typically cause in a shoe may go unrecognized. Hallux nails in this situation may develop subungual hematomas creating a negative space for microbial invasion as well as an eventual hypertrophic toenail when subject to that force chronically. Patients will often not recall the source of this nail trauma. For these patients, it is not only important to have their feet checked on a regular basis but also wear appropriate footwear that has a deep toebox and diabetic-appropriate insoles.

Nail Presentation

In a study by Al-Mutairi et al., 460 patients with diabetes and 460 patients without diabetes were evaluated. Toenails were affected in 62 % of the cases, fingernails in 23 %, and both fingernails and toenails in 14 % of the cases in the diabetic group. Distal subungual onychomycosis was found to be the most common clinical presentation seen to reflect 65 % of the patients, followed by total dystrophic onychomycosis [6]. The dominating theme was the initial presentation occurred on the feet, thus supporting the need to remove socks and shoes of those at risk for developing diabetes or are already diagnosed with in the primary physician's or specialist's office.

In most practice settings, taking a sample of the nail for fungal culture remains the gold standard when assessing pathogens of question in diabetics and nondiabetics alike. A review by Mayser et al. showed that dermatophytes are the most commonly implicated etiologic agents in diabetic and nondiabetics alike [16]. The most common agents affecting the nails are (in order) *Trichophyton rubrum* and *Trichophyton mentagrophytes var. interdigitale*, followed by *Candida* species and non-dermatophytic molds [16].

In addition to examining the diabetic patient for nail disease, it is important to examine the feet for the presence of tinea pedis. Not only can a thickened, sharp nail create a potentially serious situation but also the presence of tinea pedis that is ulcerated, fissured, or bacterially superinfected interdigitally create an equally problematic situation [15, 17]. Regarding tinea pedis, the interdigital variants, moccasin type, and vesiculobullous infection are all possible in the diabetic patient. If there is mycotic nail involvement, the practitioner should assume tinea pedis is present or will be.

Treatment

As discussed earlier, diabetic patients are particularly susceptible to fungal infections due to the modifications that occur in their immunological system; therefore, there is a need for a variety of therapies to accommodate the range of nail presentation and patient disease state [16]. Traditional treatment options for this condition include toenail debridement and drug therapies ranging from oral (terbinafine, itraconazole, fluconazole, griseofulvin) to topical (ciclopirox, efinaconazole, tavaborole) antifungal medications. However, prior to initiating antifungal therapy, it is imperative to establish a diagnosis, as other skin diseases may look similar to a fungal infection [15]. If nail mycosis is present and established, concomitant tinea pedis should be treated as well.

Nail debridement, or the process of reducing the length and thickness of a toenail, is generally a podiatric procedure. Nail debridement does make the nail cosmetically more appealing and reduces fungal load, but does not treat the fungal infection itself. It can be used as an adjunct procedure with both the oral and topical antifungals. This process not only has the potential to assist with topical therapies being more efficacious but also reduces subungual pressure and pain [15]. Regular podiatric appointments where the feet are examined and the nails are debrided can assist in preventing nail bed ulceration, especially in diabetic neuropathic patients. Certainly, in cases where the diabetic patient has neuropathy and/or retinopathy, proper foot care appointments with a specialist are key to preventing pedal complications, as nail care and inspection should be done by a medical professional. Patients absolutely should not go to a nail salon for fungal nail therapy as the instruments are not generally autoclaved which could lead to infection, and some of the toenail onychauxis is beyond what a technician can handle. With some of these problematic onychauxic nails, there are situations where a total nail avulsion may be warranted with or without nail matrix destruction to assist a patient who can't or won't use an antifungal. Prior to this procedure, vascular status should be assessed.

Matricciani et al. performed a systematic review to determine the best treatment options for diabetics who have tinea pedis or onychomycosis [17]. She and her colleagues identified six studies that evaluated the safety and efficacy of various onychomycosis treatments, but none for tinea pedis. She concluded that oral terbinafine is "as safe and effective as oral itraconazole therapy for the treatment of onychomycosis in people with diabetes" [17]. In addition to encouraging future research in tinea pedis therapies in diabetics, the systematic review found that onychomycosis cure rates in diabetics were comparable to those in nondiabetics.

One of the articles Matricciani et al. discussed determined the use of oral terbinafine in both insulin-dependent (IDDM) and non-insulin-dependent (NIDDM) diabetics [18]. Patients were administered terbinafine for 12 weeks and then followed for the duration of the study. Blood glucose levels were monitored throughout the 48-week trial. For the 89 patients who completed the trial, mycological cure was 73 %, and there was no significant difference between the IDDM and NIDDM groups. More importantly, no patients developed hypoglycemia while being treated with oral terbinafine. This is opposite of the findings of the other FDA-approved oral antifungal, itraconazole, which has been reported to increase the risk of hypoglycemia when concomitantly taking a medication from the drug classes of sulfonylurea, thiazolidinediones, or meglitinides during toenail therapy [19]. Metformin, however, does not seem to interact with the azoles, terbinafine, or griseofulvin [19]. Farkas et al. concluded that terbinafine is efficacious, tolerated, and safe when administered continuously for 12 weeks in a diabetic population [18].

Topical ciclopirox nail lacquer 8 % was the first topical antifungal approved in the USA for mild to moderate onychomycosis. In a postmarketing open-label study in Germany, ciclopirox was used in 215 diabetic patients for 6 months and was found to be safe and effective [20]. No exacerbation of diabetes or other concomitant diseases were reported during the trial. A similar trial with ciclopirox lacquer was completed in the USA with 49 patients that showed similar results in type 2 diabetic patients [21]. Armstrong et al. examined the use of topical ciclopirox and its relation to mandating daily self-inspection of the foot which could, in theory, reduce risk for a foot ulceration [22]. Seventy patients at high risk for developing a foot ulcer were followed for 12 months or until an ulcer formed. Ultimately, they didn't find an immediate prophylactic benefit to using topical ciclopirox to prevent wounds through daily foot inspection.

One of the newer topical antifungal medications, efinaconazole topical 10 % solution, showed similar complete cure (13 % diabetics vs 18.8 % nondiabetics) and mycological cure (56.5 % diabetics vs 56.3 % nondiabetics) rates in a post hoc analysis of phase 3 randomized, controlled study when comparing diabetics to nondiabetics [23]. One hundred and twelve diabetic subjects (out of 1655 total subjects) were part of this analysis, making it the largest amount of diabetics reported in a topical antifungal controlled study. Another new topical antifungal, tavaborole 5 % solution, has not reported a similar post hoc analysis, but the randomized phase 3 studies show it has a favorable benefit-risk profile in treatment of toenail onychomycosis [24]. The existence of other comorbidities, polypharmacy, and the potential for drug-drug interactions complicates the selection of an appropriate oral treatment regimen making the use of topical antifungal medications and adjunctive nail debridement a favorable choice for some of the diabetic population.

Lastly, one of the newer modalities approved to manage onychomycosis, laser therapy, has been proposed to be studied in a randomized, double-blind, controlled trial in diabetics [25]. As of this writing, the data has not been published yet; however, when completed, this would be the first double-blind laser study enrolling diabetics who are at risk for foot complications. As laser therapy is appealing to the public in its tone and connotation, an appropriate study that enrolls those with neuropathy and vascular issues could be useful when considering this modality in the future.

In conclusion, in a diabetic, the presence of mycotic nails may be a marker of atherosclerosis and lack of hyperglycemic control. Since practitioners from all specialties should be aware of the various risk factors in this patient population, the physician should have the diabetic patient remove shoes and socks during any physical examination. Treatment, not just of the nails but of any concomitant tinea pedis, should be initiated vigilantly to lessen potential lower extremity complications such as nail bed ulceration or bacterial superinfection of the interspaces, especially in the neuropathic and vascularly compromised population. Numerous treatments exist ranging from topical to oral to devices like the laser. A handful have been specifically studied in the diabetic population, but as always, it is up to the practitioner to choose the best therapy suited to their diabetic patient.

References

1. American Diabetes Association. *American Diabetes Association*. Web. 23 Feb 2016.
2. Cathcart S, Cantrell W, Elewski BE. Onychomycosis and Diabetes. JEADV. 2009;23:1119–22.
3. Elewski BE. Onychomycosis. Treatment, quality of life, and economic issues. Am J Clin Dermatol. 2000;1(1):19–26. Review
4. Dogra S, Kumar B, Bhansali A, Chakrabarty A. Epidemiology of onychomycosis in patients with diabetes mellitus in India. Int J Dermatol. 2002;41(10):647–51.

5. Gupta AK, Konnikov N, MacDonald P, Rich P, Rodger NW, Edmonds MW, McManus R, Summerbell RC. Prevalence and epidemiology of toenail onychomycosis in diabetic subjects: a multicentre survey. Br J Dermatol. 1998;139(4):665–71.
6. Al-Mutairi N, Eassa BI, Al-Rqobah DA. Clinical and mycologic characteristics of onychomycosis in diabetic patients. Acta Dermatovenerol Croat. 2010;18(2):84–91.
7. Onalan O, Adar A, Keles H, Ertugrul G, Ozkan N, Aktas H, Karakaya E. Onychomycosis is associated with subclinical atherosclerosis in patients with diabetes. Vasa. 2015;44(1):59–64.
8. Gulcan A, Gulcan E, Oksuz S, Sahin I, Kaya D. Prevalence of toenail onychomycosis in patients with type 2 diabetes mellitus and evaluation of risk factors. JAPMA. 2011;101(1):49.
9. Takehara K, Oe M, Tsunemi Y, Nagase T, Ohashi Y, Iizaka S, Ueki K, Tsukamoto K, Kadowaki T, Sanada H. Factors Associated with presence and severity of toenail onychomycosis in patients with diabetes: a cross-sectional study. Int J Nurs Stud. 2011;48:1101–8.
10. Doyle JJ, Boyko WL, Ryu S et al. Onychomycosis among diabetic patients: prevalence and impact of nonfungal foot infections. ADA 6th Annual Scientific Session; 9–13 Jun 2000; San Antonio. ADA, 2000.
11. Chang SJ, Hsu SC, Tien KJ, Hsiao JY, Lin SR, Chen HC, Hsieh MC. Metabolic syndrome associated with toenail onychomycosis in Taiwanese with diabetes mellitus. Int J Dermatol. 2008;47(5):467–72.
12. Papini M, Piraccini BM, Difonzo E, Brunoro A. Epidemiology of onychomycosis in Italy: prevalence data and risk factor identification. Mycoses. 2015;58(11):659–64. doi:10.1111/myc.12396. Epub 2015 Sep 28
13. Armstrong DG, Lavery LA, Vazquez JR, Short B, Kimbriel HR, Nixon BP, Boulton AJ. Clinical efficacy of the first metatarsophalangeal joint arthroplasty as a curative procedure for hallux interphalangeal joint wounds in patients with diabetes. Diabetes Care. 2003;26(12):3284–7.
14. Skorepová M. Mycoses and diabetes. Vnitr Lek. 2006;52(5):470–3. Review. Czech.
15. Tan JS, Joseph WS. Common fungal infections of the feet in patients with diabetes mellitus. Drugs Aging. 2004;21(2):101–12.
16. Mayser P, Freund V, Budihardja D. Toenail onychomycosis in diabetic patients. Am J Clin Dermatol. 2009;10(4):211–20.
17. Matricciani L, Talbot K, Jones S. Safety and efficacy of tinea pedis and onychomycosis treatment in people with diabetes: a systematic review. J Foot Ankle Res. 2011;4(1):26.
18. Farkas B, Paul C, Dobozy A, Hunyadi J, Horvath A, Fekete G. Terbinafine treatment of toenail onychomycosis in patients with insulin-dependent and non-insulin-dependent diabetes mellitus: a multicentre trial. Br J Dermatol. 2002;146(2):254–60.
19. Verspeelt J, Marynissen G, Gupta AK, et al. Safety of itraconazole in the diabetic population. J Am Podiatr Med Assoc. 1999;198:382–4.
20. Seebacher C, Nietsch K-H, Ulbricht HM. A multicenter, open-label study of the efficacy and safety of ciclopirox nail lacquer solution 8 % for the treatment of onychomycosis in patients with diabetes. Cutis. 2001;68:17.
21. Brenner MA, Harkless LB, Mendicino RW, Page JC. Ciclopiorx 8 % nail lacquer topical solution for the treatment of onychomycosis in patients with diabetes. J Am Podiatr Med Assoc. 2007;97(3):195–202.
22. Armstrong DV, Holtz K, Wu S. Can the use of a topical antifungal nail lacquer reduce risk for diabetic foot ulceration? Results from a randomised controlled pilot study. Int Wound J. 2005;2(2):166–70.
23. Vlahovic TC, Joseph WS. Efinaconazole topical, 10 % for the treatment of toenail onychomycosis in patients with diabetes. J Drugs Dermatol. 2014;13(10):1186–90.
24. Elewski BE, Aly R, Baldwin SL, González Soto RF, Rich P, Weisfeld M, Wiltz H, Zane LT, Pollak R. Efficacy and safety of tavaborole topical solution, 5 %, a novel boron-based antifungal agent, for the treatment of toenail onychomycosis: results from 2 randomized phase-III studies. J Am Acad Dermatol. 2015;73(1):62–9.
25. Nijenhuis-Rosien L, Kleefstra N, Wolfhagen MJ, Groenier KH, HJ B, Landman GW. Laser therapy for onychomycosis in patients with diabetes at risk for foot complications: study protocol for a randomized, double-blind, controlled trial (LASER-1). Trials. 2015;16:108.

Chapter 18
Pediatric Onychomycosis

Tracey C. Vlahovic

Prevalence

Nail conditions in children are either congenital or acquired, with the acquired conditions, like onychomycosis, appear similar, but occur with less frequency than in adults [1]. Even though nails grow at a continuous rate throughout life, the speed of growth of a pediatric nail is increased until age 10–14, where it becomes similar to that of an adult [1]. Besides the greater speed of growth in children, other thoughts as to why their nails aren't frequently as affected as adults are less exposure to higher humidity environments, less trauma due to a smaller nail surface area, and lower incidence of the often concomitant tinea pedis [2]. Even with these facts, onychomycosis is one of the most common nail diseases in the pediatric population, with adolescents being affected more than younger children.

The literature concurs that pediatric onychomycosis is less common than in adults (0.3 % vs 2–13 %), but its existence is starting to rise [3]. Plausible causes for pediatric onychomycosis to be increasing include the presence of genetic predisposition to developing the dermatophyte infection in the presence of an affected family member, juvenile diabetes, Down's syndrome, immunocompromised disorders such as a transplant recipient and HIV, and lifestyle issues as increased wearing of occlusive shoe gear [4]. In addition to these, other risk factors to developing onychomycosis in a child are living in a rural area, hypoxemia, metabolic alterations, repetitive trauma, and malignant neoplasms [2]. A study of 72 children, ages 2–18 years old, at an oncology clinic in Mexico, showed the frequency of onychomycosis in this immunosuppressed population as one child or 1.3 % [2]. The authors theorized that the frequency of nail mycosis in this immunosuppressed population wasn't greater than average due to the almost protective benefits of pediatric nail growth (not allowing dermatophytes to colonize due to the rapid growth) and possibly the cytotoxic

T.C. Vlahovic, DPM, FFPM RCPS (Glasg)
Department of Podiatric Medicine, Temple University School of Podiatric Medicine,
148 N 8th Street, Philadelphia, 19107 PA, USA
e-mail: traceyv@temple.edu

A. Tosti et al. (eds.), *Onychomycosis*, DOI 10.1007/978-3-319-44853-4_18

effect of the chemotherapeutic agents the children were exposed to [2]. In this particular population, the lack of increased nail mycosis does not mean they won't have a susceptibility to disseminated fungal infections and certainly should be examined for such.

As in adults, the most common type of onychomycosis seen in children is the distal lateral subungual type, but proximal subungual and superficial white types can occur with less frequency [4]. Both the deep and classic types of superficial white occur more in younger children [1]. Candida onychomycosis is rare but, if present, coexists with a paronychia [4]. The total dystrophic type is the rarest in children. In a review of 59 cases of pediatric onychomycosis in children 0–18, 66.1 % had toenail versus fingernail onychomycosis with distal lateral subungual being the most common type [5]. The older children were the highest cohort to see mycotic nails, with a male predilection [5]. In agreement with the literature, the most common dermatophyte, *Trichophyton rubrum*, affects the nail the most; followed by *C. albicans*, *C. parapsilosis*, and *C. tropicalis* [5–7]. Interestingly, 14 of the 59 children had concomitant tinea pedis, and eight of the parents of these children had either tinea pedis or onychomycosis [5]. In another review of 16 cases of nail mycosis in children under the age of 2, Bonifaz et al. found the majority with distal subungual onychomycosis had Down's syndrome, with one having concomitant tinea capitis and two being preterm [8]. Although not a common risk factor, preterm children have shorter nail plates which may account for this increased prevalence [8].

As in adults, dermatophytes can produce pigmentation that may appear as a melanocytic lesion. Besides completing a thorough history and physical, it is important to get mycological confirmation as onychomycosis in a child may mimic various nail issues. Differential diagnoses of onychomycosis in a child would include the following: trauma, psoriasis, lichen planus, alopecia areata, atopic dermatitis, various congenital nail disorders, and nevi [4]. As described in previous chapters, a specimen for fungal culture should be submitted prior to starting any antifungal therapy. Wiping the nail with alcohol prior to trimming the nail back to the mycelial front (the area of subungual activity), and then obtaining the hyperkeratotic subungual material, is what is best for specimen collection [4].

Choosing the Best Treatment

As with an adult, consideration of the patient age, nail involvement, pathogen, drug-drug interactions, and medical history are factors when choosing a treatment plan. As of this writing, there are no FDA-approved treatments for pediatric onychomycosis. In time, this might change as there is a phase IV efinaconazole 10 % solution trial involving children underway and a new oral antifungal, VT-1161, which is being investigated for a range of fungal diseases, including onychomycosis. That said, most practitioners will prescribe oral or topical antifungal therapy for children, while some might choose avulsion, laser, or other medical devices even though there is no evidence to support their pediatric use [9].

Systemic Antifungals

In their meta-analysis of systemic antifungal use in children under the age of 18, Gupta and Paquet showed a complete cure rate of 70.8 % when systemic antifungals were solely used [3]. This complete cure rate was increased to 80.0 % with the addition of a topical antifungal in several cases [3]. Ultimately, terbinafine, itraconazole, fluconazole, and griseofulvin had safety and efficacy profiles similar to those reported for adults [3].

As with adults, systemic antifungals are generally chosen where 50 % of the distal nail plate is affected, multiple nails are involved, and topical therapy may not be useful. With a mycological cure of 70 % in toenails, terbinafine is FDA approved for tinea capitis in children but is off-label for pediatric onychomycosis. That said, the adult dose of 250 mg daily in an adult is not recommended in children weighing less than 40 kg. The pediatric dosage regimen is as follows: 62.5 mg for children weighing less than 20 kg, 125 mg in those weighing between 20 and 40 kg, and 250 mg in those who weigh greater than 40 kg. Besides being available as a tablet, it is also available as an oral granule, which is helpful in children who are unable to swallow pills. In adults, the complete cure rate for terbinafine is 38 % in toenails, but in a systematic review in its use in children, a pooled complete cure rate of 78.8 % has been reported [3]. Adverse events seen in the pediatric population when taking terbinafine have included acute urticaria, anorexia, tiredness, vesiculopustular eruption, and agranulocytosis [3]. As in adults, the measurement of AST and ALT is recommended before starting this therapy in a child, and of course, dispensing of this medication in those with pre-existing liver disease should be avoided.

A broad spectrum antifungal, itraconazole is available as a suspension and as an oral capsule which is useful in children who can't tolerate swallowing pills. Like terbinafine, the dosing for a child is weight based: 5 mg/kg/day in those weighing less than 50 kg and those who weigh more than 50 kg may receive the adult dose of 200 mg/day [9]. If administering the capsule to a child, it should be ingested after a full meal [6]. In contrast, the itraconazole oral solution which may be given as a dose of 3 mg/kg/day should be given under fasting conditions [6, 10]. Adult studies have shown better efficacy in pulse dosing than continuous dosing of itraconazole. In children, the opposite has been observed with a systematic review reporting a complete cure rate of 68.4 % for the pulse dosing versus 87.7 % for the continuous dosing regimen [3]. Due to the drug-drug interactions and adverse events, itraconazole is not often the best choice for adults. In children, due to their lack of systemic conditions and medication use that can potentially interact with itraconazole, the adverse events are mild and include fatigue, gastrointestinal symptoms, and headache [3]. Liver function studies should also be performed prior to initiating itraconazole therapy in a child.

Approved in Europe for onychomycosis, but off-label in the USA, fluconazole with its once weekly dosing until the nail grows out requires longer therapy than either itraconazole or terbinafine. This could range between 9 and 18 months for toenail onychomycosis [9]. Available as a tablet or an oral suspension, fluconazole is not often used as first-line therapy; however, in a meta-analysis of its use in children, the complete cure was reported as 66.7 % [9]. The dosage for children ranges from 3 to 6 mg/kg/day in either a continuous or pulse dose regimen [10]. In children, the adverse advents possible when taking fluconazole are abdominal pain, rash, renal dysfunction, nausea, vomiting, and diarrhea. Another systemic antifungal, griseofulvin, has also been reported as a therapy for onychomycosis and like fluconazole is administered until the nail grows out fully, but reported cure rates are low [10].

Topical Antifungals

In the USA, ciclopirox 8 % lacquer, efinaconazole 10 % topical solution, and tavaborole 5 % topical solution have been approved for topical onychomycosis therapy. In Europe, there is also the addition of topical amorolfine 5 % nail lacquer [9]. These medications can be used as stand-alone therapies or in conjunction with oral therapy and/or nail debridement. Most parents prefer the use of a topical therapy for their child as they feel it is safer and are worried about their child ingesting a tablet. Certainly, an aversion to taking an oral medication would be a reason to use a topical over an oral in this population, but other factors such as nail involvement, number of nails involved, and predisposing medical history should also be considered.

Since children have thin, fast-growing nails, topical therapy is well suited for this population. Topical therapy still requires once-daily application but is possible to have a decreased treatment period due to the nature of their nail growth [9].

Currently, ciclopirox is the only topical antifungal that has been evaluated for the safety and efficacy of onychomycosis in a clinical trial involving children [11]. In this randomized, double-blind, vehicle-controlled trial involving 40 children from 2 to 16 years old, 92 % of those who had a clinical cure remained clear after 1 year. At 32 weeks, 77 % of those who received ciclopirox had a mycological cure [11]. Numerous case reports in the literature have described the use of ciclopirox for congenital candidiasis of the fingernail, white superficial onychomycosis, and *T. rubrum* that caused distal subungual onychomycosis [9].

The other topical antifungals have not been formally approved for use in children, but studies and case reports have shown their usefulness. Regarding the use of amorolfine in children, there have been two case studies that involved a child with white superficial onychomycosis and another child with distal subungual onychomycosis of the fingernail. Both achieved some level of improvement in a faster treatment time than an adult [9]. As of this writing, there is a phase IV study examining efinaconazole 10 % solution in children ages 6–16 years [12]. No pediatric studies have been initiated with tavaborole 5 % solution at this time.

Other Therapies

Surgical avulsion has been reported as a therapy for onychomycosis in adults, but no formal studies have been performed on children involving this modality. Chemical avulsion, utilizing a urea compound, to soften and initiate nontraumatic removal of the nail has been reported in children. In a study involving 25 children under 16 years old, a urea ointment was applied to chemically avulse the nail followed by a topical antifungal applied to the nail bed. After 4 weeks of topical antifungal therapy to the nail unit area, 17 children achieved "cure," six improved, and two failed therapy [9, 13]. Other device-based modalities such as laser and photodynamic therapy have been used in adults but not yet studied in children.

Conclusion

Even though this nail disease occurs less in children than in adults, it is important to understand the pathogenesis, treatment, and risks/benefits of various therapeutic modalities when treating pediatric onychomycosis. Recurrence of nail disease may occur as the child grows older, has a genetic predisposition, develops tinea pedis, has a comorbid state-like diabetes, is immunocompromised, and wears occlusive footwear. Screening of other family members for both onychomycosis and tinea pedis may lessen recurrence, but ultimately the diligent use of antifungal therapy plays a large role in obtaining treatment success. Noncompliance in a pediatric population can be frustrating when the child refuses treatment by the parent and is expected and fails to apply treatment him/herself or the parents themselves do not comply with the treatment regimen for the child. Education of the parent and child on onychomycosis regarding what to expect, how to take/apply prescribed therapy, and the length of therapy is key. Besides pharmacological agents, appropriate foot hygiene, shoe and sock changes, and observation of signs and symptoms of skin dermatophytosis should be reviewed and implemented into the patient's environment.

Many of the available oral and topical therapies that have been studied in adults have shown to be safe and efficacious in children in a limited amount of published studies. Oral therapies have proven to be beneficial in the pediatric population, but future studies with the newer topical agents may prove the same advantage. Ultimately, careful monitoring for nail growth with the selected antifungal agent and education of the family on the chosen therapy along with environmental changes in the pediatric population is paramount to achieve the mycological and visually clear nail that is desired by the practitioner and the patient.

References

1. Piraccini BM, Starace M. Nail disorders in infants and children. Curr Opin Pediatr. 2014; 26(4):440–5.
2. García-Romero MT, Lopez-Aguilar E, Arenas R. Onychomycosis in immunosuppressed children receiving chemotherapy. Pediatr Dermatol. 2014;31(5):618–20. doi:10.1111/pde.12030. Epub 2012 Oct 29.
3. Gupta AK, Paquet M. Systemic antifungals to treat onychomycosis in children: a systematic review. Pediatr Dermatol. 2013;30(3):294–302. Epub 2012 Dec 26.
4. Chu DH, Rubin AI. Diagnosis and management of nail disorders in children. Pediatr Clin N Am. 2014;61(2):293–308. Epub 2014 Jan 21.

5. Kim DM, Suh MK, Ha GY. Onychomycosis in children: an experience of 59 cases. Ann Dermatol. 2013;25(3):327–34. Epub 2013 Aug 13.
6. Gupta AK, Skinner AR, Baran R. Onychomycosis in children: an overview. J Drugs Dermatol. 2003;2(1):31–4.
7. Young LS, Arbuckle HA, Morelli JG. Onychomycosis in the Denver pediatrics population, a retrospective study. Pediatr Dermatol. 2014;31(1):106–8. Epub 2012 May 21.
8. Bonifaz A, Saúl A, Mena C, Valencia A, Paredes V, Fierro L, Araiza J. Dermatophyte onychomycosis in children under 2 years of age: experience of 16 cases. J Eur Acad Dermatol Venereol. 2007;21(1):115–7.
9. Feldstein S, Totri C, Friedlander SF. Antifungal therapy for onychomycosis in children. Clin Dermatol. 2015;33(3):333–9. Epub 2014 Dec 8.
10. Ginter-Hanselmayer G, Weger W, Smolle J. Onychomycosis: a new emerging infectious disease in childhood population and adolescents. Report on treatment experience with terbinafine and itraconazole in 36 patients. J Eur Acad Dermatol Venereol. 2008;22(4):470–5.
11. Friedlander SF, Chan YC, Chan YH, Eichenfeld LF. Onychomycosis does not always require systemic treatment for a cure: a trial using topical therapy. Pediatr Dermatol. 2013;30:316–22.
12. Safety and pharmacokinetics of Efinaconazole Topical Solution in subjects with mild to severe onychomycosis. https://clinicaltrials.gov/ct2/show/NCT02812771.
13. Bonifaz A, Ibarra G. Onychomycosis in children: treatment with bifonazole-urea. Pediatr Dermatol. 2000;17:310–4.

Chapter 19
The Podiatric Approach

Tracey C. Vlahovic

Podiatric physicians have a unique practice situation, as they generally manage onychomycosis cases on a daily basis and in a specialized population (diabetes, Chap. 17). However, toenail disease may be caused by a variety of issues that are specifically foot related and not fungal related: trauma from shoes, biomechanical issues and forces, and infection compounded by shoe gear and adjacent skin conditions to the nails (i.e., interdigital tinea pedis). It is important when discussing the management and treatment of toenail onychomycosis that the visually similar biomechanical causes of nail dystrophy are also mentioned.

Patients commonly present to a podiatric physician's office for the care of toenail pain (both infectious and noninfectious causes), discoloration that is cosmetically displeasing, and/or thickness that creates pressure in shoes. Patients are often under the belief that their nail presentation may be the result of a fungal infection; however, it is imperative that other factors on and around the nail unit are considered: biomechanics and shoe gear. These are unique to the toenail when compared to the fingernail. Biomechanics describes both the non-pathological and pathological forces involved in the gait cycle. The pathologic forces may result in digital deformities, soft tissue lesions (i.e., corns and calluses), bunions, arch and heel pain, and even skin breakdown (especially in a neuropathic patient). Both in the diabetic neuropathic population and those with painful or biomechanical issues, the podiatric practitioner will likely perform a biomechanical evaluation which includes gait analysis and function of the major joints of the foot and ankle.

T.C. Vlahovic, DPM, FFPM RCPS (Glasg)
Department of Podiatric Medicine, Temple University School of Podiatric Medicine, 148 N 8th St, Philadelphia, 19107 PA, USA
e-mail: traceyv@temple.edu

A. Tosti et al. (eds.), *Onychomycosis*, DOI 10.1007/978-3-319-44853-4_19

Evaluating the Podiatric Patient

To evaluate a patient presenting with toenail onychomycosis, the practitioner should begin with completing a thorough history and physical evaluation. With treatment options ranging from systemic to surgical, knowledge of medical history, current medications, and family history will aid differential diagnosis and treatment plan. Key questions include how long have you had the nail changes, is it painful, and has it affected your quality of life? Is the patient able to bend and visualize the nails in order to trim them? Daily shoe gear choices, work and athletic activities, and home and work environment will all assist treatment plan selection. Level of immunosuppression, pedal vascular status, and ability to take oral or apply topical medication should be taken into account. Discussion and examination of any other skin rashes or conditions should be completed, as psoriasis and eczema can mimic mycotic toenails.

Visual assessment is imperative. Since the Zaias classification was proposed in 1972, modifications have been proposed and published to reflect the wide array of dermatophytes, non-dermatophyte molds, and yeasts as well as the complications of various patterns occurring in the same nail or other inflammatory diseases co-presenting with mycosis [1]. Nail plate changes include:

- DLSO where the invasion begins at the hyponychium and disturbs the distal nail bed
- Proximal subungual onychomycosis (PSO) where invasion begins proximally
- Superficial white onychomycosis (SWO) where the upper surface of the nail plate is first attacked [1]
- Total dystrophic which describes total nail plate involvement and surrounding periungual tissue
- Endonyx onychomycosis (EO) which describes distal nail plate attack resulting in a deeper penetration of hyphae

In addition, the physician should determine how many toenails are involved on one or both feet, percent involvement of the nail, any biomechanically aggravating factors that could contribute to nail dystrophy (adductovarus fifth digit, hammertoe, or hallux valgus), and the presence of tinea pedis interdigitally or plantarly.

Approximately 50 % of nail disease is caused by onychomycosis [2]; the remainder conditions mimic onychomycosis, having similar signs and symptoms including psoriasis, lichen planus, reactive arthritis, allergic/irritant contact dermatitis, and eczema. Other differential diagnoses include alopecia, nail changes secondary to biomechanical issues, melanoma (and other skin cancers), traumatic onycholysis, 20-nail dystrophy, and pachyonychia [3–5].

Since not all presenting nail disease is mycotic, it is important to confirm with laboratory diagnosis if the treatment plan includes oral antifungal therapy, if there is concomitant skin disease difficult to distinguish in the nails, and if the patient has been on antifungal therapy previously and disease has recurred. Laboratory diagnostic methods include direct microscopy (KOH test), nail plate biopsy for periodic acid-Schiff

(PAS) stain, and fungal culture. Generally, KOH and fungal culture are done together; KOH shows the presence of hyphae and cultures the species present. Unfortunately, fungal cultivation is a slow process (up to 4 weeks) and may generate false-negative results in 40 % of the cases that are microscopically positive [6]. An alternative PAS involves sending nail plate (commonly referred to as, but not a true biopsy) for staining to determine presence of dermatophytes. PAS provides quicker results and is more sensitive, while culture is the more specific (regarding species) [7–9].

Standard mycological tests, KOH and fungal culture, may yield false-negative or false-positive results, and require time to verify the pathogens [10]. Accurate diagnoses are often delayed due to lack of both specific and rapid methods of pathogen identification. When the mycological analyses are negative and clinical picture highly suggestive of onychomycosis, polymerase chain reaction (PCR) testing may be an option [11]. Antifungal drug efficacy and dosages may differ for different causative pathogens, and it has been hypothesized that mixed and non-dermatophyte onychomycosis may be cause for high rate of treatment failures [12]. A rapidly sensitive method for detection and identification will better guide an appropriate treatment strategy. PCR detects a specific DNA sequence; moreover, fungi species-specific PCR diagnostic methods are available deepening our understanding and treatment of onychomycosis [13–15]. Since DNA is extremely resistant and can persist even in the absence of viable hyphae, DNA amplification techniques such as PCR may represent a useful addition to standard procedure [16]. Time will tell how truly beneficial PCR will be both in the physician office and in clinical trials.

Podiatric Nail Issues

Toenail Onychomycosis

Onychomycosis or tinea unguium is caused by invasion of the nail unit by dermatophytes, non-dermatophyte molds, and/or *Candida albicans*. Toenails subject to trauma from either a biomechanical reason or otherwise may be the first to present. For example, a limitation in plantarflexory motion of the first metatarsophalangeal joint may predispose the hallux nail to trauma against the toe box of the shoe, thus allowing dermatophyte invasion to take place. In addition to nail trauma as a harbinger of mycosis, tinea pedis or tinea cruris on the patient may be concomitantly found and be a source of infection. When a patient presents with mycotic toenails, it is useful not only to inspect interdigitally and plantarly for signs of tinea pedis but also to ask if they have any scaly rashes elsewhere on the body or past use of a topical antifungal anywhere else on the body.

Podiatric practitioners recommend the oral and topical medications and laser procedures that have been covered in this book (Chaps 19, 20, and 21). Some podiatric physicians recommend in-office-dispensed, over-the-counter, and compounded topical remedies as a convenience and cost-saving entity to the patients; however, these are not specifically FDA approved for mycotic toenails. Also, topical urea preparations have classically been used to soften, thin, and smooth the nail plate both before and during topical antifungal therapy but have not been specifically studied in a clinical trial.

One of the most common podiatric in-office procedures, nail debridement, is defined as the mechanical reduction of toenail length and thickness using nail nipper or rotating burr (such as a Dremel device). Nail debridement may provide a valuable adjunct for patients experiencing pain upon ambulation and in shoe gear [17]. While debridement alone improves quality of life and nail thickness, it does not result in mycological cure [18]. In one study, the concomitant use of topical ciclopirox and debridement improved a patient's quality of life and resulted in mycologic cure [18]. However, debridement added to oral antifungal therapy may offer a only a small benefit [19, 20]. Debridement can provide pain relief and improved patient satisfaction, affording an opportunity to encourage adherence. It may offer benefits through reduced fungal load and enhanced penetration of topical drugs into the nail unit. For patients who opt against pharmacological treatment, debridement will allow more comfort in shoe gear and reduce potential pressure on the nail bed, especially if diabetic neuropathy is present. In the diabetic patient who is compromised both vascularly and neurologically, mycotic nail debridement is routinely performed by a podiatric practitioner every 9–12 weeks in order to decrease pressure and complications that may arise from the thickness of nails and prevent the patient from creating a problematic situation by performing self-care of the nails.

Nail avulsion, a procedure that creates separation of the nail plate from the nail bed, can be achieved nonsurgically with daily application of topical 40 % urea for 1–2 weeks [21]. Generally, this is followed by application of a topical antifungal once the toenail has been removed, repeating as necessary. It is more common in Europe [21]. Chemical nail avulsion can be useful in patients who have a needle/procedure phobia, who have peripheral vascular disease or another comorbidity precluding pharmacological intervention, or have a single nail infected. However, removal of the nail itself will not result in clearance of the infection, even followed by topical antifungal therapy.

For a singularly painful or thickened nail, some patients may opt for a surgical total nail removal. Surgery involves application of local anesthesia to the digit followed by removal of the nail plate in toto. Simple total avulsion of the nail itself is not curative for a mycotic nail; as the procedure has not addressed the basis of infection. Combining nail avulsion and topical antifungals has been described as the preferred treatment plan. Total nail avulsion with the use of a topical azole cream applied twice daily to the exposed nail bed resulted in a high dropout rate. All patients with total dystrophic onychomycosis failed, and only 56 % patients (15/27) were cured with this approach suggesting that the procedure should not be generally suggested for the treatment of onychomycosis [22].

Nail avulsion has been suggested to obtain a better specimen for fungal culture but should only be used in situations where both systemic and topical antifungal therapies have failed [21]. Contraindications include patients with peripheral vascular disease, autoimmune disorders, collagen vascular disease, diabetes, hemostasis disorders, and acute infection/inflammation of the periungual tissue [23]. Possible keratinization of the nail bed as the nail plate is growing is also a concern, thus creating a "disappearing nail bed" scenario where the nail plate will never adhere to the nail bed [24].

Mimickers of Toenail Onychomycosis: General Toenail Onychodystrophy

Toenail appearance and discomfort in shoe gear are the main motivators for most patients to schedule a podiatric consultation. During that patient visit, it is important for the practitioner to delve into the cause of the problematic toenail change, generally known as onychodystrophy. Onychodystrophy, which is any alteration of nail morphology, encompasses a wide spectrum of nail disorders [25]. Caused by either exogenous or endogenous factors, nail dystrophy may manifest as a misshapen, damaged, infected, or discolored nail unit that may affect the fingernails, toenails, or both.

Morphologic terms commonly used to describe these affected nails are onycholysis, onychauxis, and onychorrhexis. Onycholysis is separation of the nail plate from the nail bed and may be caused by exogenous trauma, but also may be caused by a systemic disorder like psoriasis. The pocket created also creates a pathway for dermatophytes to infect the nail bed. According to Bodman, it is caused by repetitive microtrauma, which can be caused by ill-fitting shoe gear and subsequent nail unit impingement [26]. As he notes, this commonly occurs not only in longer toes but also in the hallucal and fifth toenails especially in "slip-on shoes that hug the heels and grab the toes to stay on the foot." One may also see onycholysis in patients who have hallux limitus and compensate by increased motion in the hallux interphalangeal joint, which ultimately causes impingement of the nail against the toe box. Distal onycholysis may be seen in patients who chronically get pedicures as a result of the instrument trauma during that salon service.

Onychauxis is thickening of the nail unit seen both in onychomycosis and psoriasis. Onychorrhexis presents as nail plate ridges parallel to the lateral nail fold. This may be seen as a sign of normal aging or as the manifestation of underlying diseases such as lichen planus and psoriasis [27]. Beau's lines are depressions that run transversely across the nail plate. The width of the depression correlates with the length of the insult to the proximal nail matrix [25]. Beau's lines can occur singly (one event or illness) or with multiple bands (multiple repeated trauma). I see this nail manifestation in people who chronically get pedicures, those who play basketball or tennis (or any sport that stops and starts with the nails hitting the front of the shoe), and those who wear tight-fitting shoes and clogs.

Onychatrophia is a condition which typically occurs in the fifth toes and is a size and thickness reduction of the nail plate. Onychatrophia may be caused by shoe-induced microtrauma, and other causes include peripheral vascular disease or lichen planus. The condition also may have a congenital origin.

In the office, when patients have presented with these onychodystrophies, the patient usually feels the affected nail is onychomycotic. While onycholysis can be the starting point for onychomycosis, Beau's lines can occur in fungal nails, and onychatrophia on the fifth toes may appear similar to nail fungus. It is important for the practitioner to distinguish between these traumatically induced deformities of the nail unit and true dermatophyte infection.

The most common type of nail dystrophy seen by podiatric practitioners is onychomycosis which represents about half of the pathologies seen [25], but the physician should be aware of the numerous other pathologies that may mimic dermatophyte infection of the nail such as psoriasis, lichen planus, trachyonychia, and trauma.

Trauma-Induced Onychodystrophy

Trauma can manifest in various ways to the toenails: exogenous means and secondary to the unique skeletal construct of the digit.

During a pedicure, the process of manipulating the cuticle may lead to Beau's lines, or depressions of the nail plate that are parallel to the proximal nail fold. Also, scraping of the hyponychium can lead to onycholysis which provides a pocket for dermatophyte infection to take hold.

Often due to shoe gear and the shape and direction of the fifth digit, the fifth toenail often becomes dystrophic and thickened [26]. Patients and practitioners alike will confuse this with onychomycosis. If one sees this with concomitant onychomycosis and treats the patient systemically, the practitioner should discuss with the patient the possibility that the fifth toenail may not respond to oral or topical antifungals. The underlying cause of the dystrophy can be biomechanical (adductovarus fifth toe where the digit is externally rotated and the nail is parallel to the side of the shoe) or tight-fitting shoes. A Lister's corn or focal hyperkeratotic lesion that may appear to the patient as a "split nail" lateral to the nail plate may also be present.

Onychauxis, onycholysis, and discoloration secondary to the trauma of a severely contracted hammertoe may frustrate the patient who is pursuing antifungal therapy and questioning why a treatment regimen is not successful. In these cases, it is imperative to educate the patient about the biomechanical cause of the nail thickening and the treatment options which range from purchasing a shoe with a deeper toe box to decrease pressure to surgical management of the digital deformity if warranted.

Ambulation Disorders/Biomechanical Problems

As the armor protecting the distal phalanx is being subjected to aforementioned daily trauma from shoe gear and biomechanical forces during the gait cycle, the toenail can experience pathologies that run the gamut from hematoma to infection.

Asymmetrical Gait Nail Unit Syndrome

Zaias described a clinical entity where one hallux nail is dystrophic or onycholytic and the other nine are fairly normal in appearance. This lone dystrophic nail looks like onychomycosis and has failed all conservative and surgical methods which has resulted in patient frustration. This solo nail pathology may be asymmetric gait nail unit syndrome or AGNUS [28].

Due to performing gait analysis and clinically observing asymmetrical pathology, podiatric physicians especially understand the body is not symmetrical, even when it comes to toenails. As described earlier, faulty biomechanics can affect the nail. AGNUS combines the biomechanical aspect with the notion that the feet aren't mirror images. AGNUS is simply defined as "dermatophyte fungus-negative abnormal nail as a result of toe friction in a closed shoe in patients with asymmetrical walking gait" [28, 29]. It begins with a unilateral hallux nail presentation but may eventually involve both halluces. Patients may also complain of back pain. Ultimately, these nails look onychomycotic but are frequently fungal culture negative. There is onycholysis distally, may have hyperkeratosis at the tip of the toe, and, as Zaias describes it, asymmetrical walking gait due to dysfunctional foot biomechanics (which he ascertained by looking at shoe wear patterns). The nails might look more opaque or discolored than the non-affected nails. He hypothesized that the friction of the shoe against the nail in a patient with abnormal gait will lead to AGNUS. Therefore, part of his treatment regimen is to have the patient forgo closed-toed shoes.

In this author's experience, patients who fit this description improved in the summer months when they could wear open-toed shoes daily. However, all of those positive changes regressed once they returned to closed-toed shoes in the fall and winter months. Beyond recommending wearing open-toed shoes for the majority of the year, the physician has to determine what the optimal treatment biomechanically may be like insoles, deep toe box shoes, or accommodative lycra toe box-based shoes that would give with each step. These modalities have not been assessed specifically for AGNUS, and further research will need to be completed in this area.

Other Nail Pathologies Caused by Biomechanical Issues

Hallux valgus or the bunion deformity is the rotation and abductory movement of the great toe toward the second toe. This results in a hypertrophic dorsal-medial eminence at the first metatarsal which may or may not be painful. The hallux may underlap or overlap the second digit or abut closely to it. This may result in the following nail pathologies: hypertrophic nail plate, onychocryptosis, subungual hematoma, and onycholysis (which may lead to onychomycosis). Onychocryptosis may occur on either the medial or lateral hallux nail margin. If accompanied by erythema, edema, and granulation tissue, a partial nail avulsion is warranted. However, it should be noted that this entity may return if the underlying hallux valgus deformity is not addressed. A functional orthotic device with or without a surgical procedure where the hallux and metatarsal are brought back into alignment are treatment choices for this nail issue as well as the others mentioned. A deeper toe box and nail debridement are additional conservative options to both biomechanical assistance and surgical correction.

Hallux limitus/rigidus describes a condition where there is jamming of the proximal phalanx on the first metatarsal resulting in the loss of range of motion in the dorsiflexion motion. This is accompanied by increased motion in the interphalangeal joint to accommodate for the lack of motion at the first metatarsophalangeal joint. This results in the hallux nail being in a more dorsiflexed position and repetitive trauma of the nail against the top of the toe box. The hallux nail can become thickened or onycholytic and predispose the nail unit to a dermatophyte infection. Conservative methods include debriding the nail and functional orthotics. Surgical procedure involves manipulation of the first metatarsal or fusion of the first metatarsophalangeal joint to bring the first ray back into alignment. Ultimately, this would affect the nail unit in a positive manner.

Contracted digits or hammertoes are a result of multiple forces in the foot that causes the digits to buckle at the proximal interphalangeal joint or the distal interphalangeal joint. The toenail is pointing downward in these cases and is subjected to constant repetitive microtrauma from the ground and sole of the shoe. The nail becomes onychauxic and onycholytic which may predispose it to dermatophyte infection. The nail may also be devoid of fungal infection and appears hypertrophic simply as a response to the constant trauma. Conservative measures include nail debridement, orthodigital devices to take pressure off the distal tip of the toe, and a deeper toe box shoe. Surgical methods include an invasive procedure to straighten the toe by performing an arthroplasty to the contracted joint in question.

The adductovarus fifth toe presents as a rotated digit where the patient is walking on the lateral aspect of the toenail. There is often focal hyperkeratotic tissue that resembles a toenail lateral to the nail plate that appears as a "split" nail. Also, there might be a hyperkeratotic lesion (corn) on the proximal interphalangeal joint that is a source for pain in shoe gear. The fifth toenail may become hyperkeratotic and painful. This may visually look identical to onychomycosis but rarely is dermatophyte infected [30]. Shoe gear and biomechanics are the major causes of this nail pathology. A wider toe box shoe and orthotics may be helpful along with nail debridement, but many of these patients will go on to have a surgical procedure to derotate the fifth digit.

Conclusion

For most podiatric practitioners, the care and management of toenail onychomycosis is a large part of a medical practice. It is not only important for a podiatric practitioner to collaborate with other medical specialties when treating a patient for this entity but also prudent for non-podiatrists to realize the spectrum of toenail disease that can be caused by daily external forces. Due to shoe gear, mechanical forces from the ground and gait, and body weight in general, the toenails are subject to deforming forces that may result in nail pathology. They are a unique entity that shouldn't be assessed simply by their visual presence but also by the exogenous factors they are being faced with in daily life.

References

1. Hay RJ, Baran R. Onychomycosis: A proposed revision of the clinical classification. J Am Acad Dermatol. 2011;65:1219–27.
2. Faergemann J, Baran R. Epidemiology, clinical presentation and diagnosis of onychomycosis. Br J Dermatol. 2003;149(Suppl):1–4.
3. Murphy F, Jiaravuthisan MM, Sasseville D, et al. Psoriasis of the nail: anatomy, pathology, clinical presentation, and review of the literature on therapy. J Am Acad Dermatol. 2007;57(1):1–27.
4. Rich P, Elewski B, Scher RK, et al. Diagnosis, clinical implications, and complications of onychomycosis. Semin Cutan Med Surg. 2013;32(2Suppl 1):S5–8.
5. Moll JM. Seronegative arthropathies in the foot. Baillieres Clin Rheumatol. 1987;1(2): 289–314.
6. Fletcher CL, Hay RJ, Smeeton NC. Onychomycosis: the development of a clinical diagnostic aid for toenail disease. Part I. Establishing discriminating historical and clinical features. Br J Dermatol. 2004;150:701–5.
7. Weinberg JM, Koestenblatt EK, Tutrone WD, et al. Comparison of diagnostic methods in the evaluation of onychomycosis. J Am Acad Dermatol. 2003;49(2):193–7.
8. Reisberger E-M, Abels C, Landthaler M, et al. Histopathological diagnosis of onychomycosis by periodic acid-Schiff-stained nail clippings. Br J Dermatol. 2003;148(4):749–54.
9. Borkowski P, Williams M, Holewinski J, et al. Onychomycosis: an analysis of 50 cases and a comparison of diagnostic techniques. J Am Podiatr Med Assoc. 2001;91(7):351–5.
10. Elewski BE. Diagnostic techniques for confirming onychomycosis. J Am Acad Dermatol. 1996;35:56–60.
11. Arca E, Saracli MA, Akar A, et al. Polymerase chain reaction in the diagnosis of onychomycosis. Eur J Dermatol. 2004;14:52–5.
12. Pierard GE, Arrese-Estrada J, Pierard-Franchimont C. Treatment of onychomycosis: traditional approaches. J Am Acad Dermatol. 1993;29:S41–5.
13. Spreadbury C, Holden D, Aufaurre-Brown A, et al. Detection of aspergillus fumigatus by polymerase chain reaction. J Clin Microbiol. 1993;31:615–21.
14. Miyakawa Y, Mabuchi T, Kagaya K, et al. Isolation and characterization of a species-specific DNA fragment for detection of *Candida albicans* by polymerase chain reaction. J Clin Microbiol. 1992;30:894–900.
15. Baharaeen S, Vishniac HS. 25S ribosomal RNA homologies of basidiomycetous yeasts: taxonomic and phylogenetic implications. Can J Microbiol. 1984;30:613–21.
16. Walberg M, Mørk C, Sandven P, et al. 18S rDNA polymerase chain reaction and sequencing in onychomycosis diagnostics. Acta Derm Venereol. 2006;86:223–6.
17. Potter LP, Mathias SD, Raut M, et al. The impact of aggressive debridement used as an adjunct therapy with terbinafine on perceptions of patients undergoing treatment for toenail onychomycosis. J Dermatolog Treat. 2007;18:46–52.
18. Malay DS, Yi S, Borowsky P, et al. Efficacy of debridement alone versus debridement combined with topical antifungal nail lacquer for the treatment of pedal onychomycosis: a randomized, controlled trial. J Foot Ankle Surg. 2009;48:294–308.

19. Jennings MB, Pollak R, Harkless LB, et al. Treatment of toenail onychomycosis with oral terbinafine plus aggressive debridement: IRON-CLAD, a large, randomized, open-label, multicenter trial. J Am Podiatr Med Assoc. 2006;96:465–73.
20. Vlahovic TC, Joseph WS, Scher RK, Tosti A, Plasencia J, Pariser DM, Markinson BC. Diagnosis and management of onychomycosis: perspectives from a joint podiatry-dermatology roundtable. J Am Podiatr Med Assoc. 2016;106(2):155–62.
21. Gupta AK, Paquet M, Simpson FC. Therapies for the treatment of onychomycosis. Clin Dermatol. 2013;31(5):544–54.
22. Grover C, Bansal S, Nanda S, et al. Combination of surgical avulsion and topical therapy for single nail onychomycosis: a randomized controlled trial. Br J Dermatol. 2007;157(2):364–8.
23. Pandhi D, Verma P. Nail avulsion: Indications and methods (surgical nail avulsion). Indian J Dermatol Venereol Leprol. 2012;78:299–308.
24. Daniel CR 3rd, Tosti A, Iorizzo M, Piraccini BM. The disappearing nail bed: a possible outcome of onycholysis. Cutis. 2005;76(5):325–7.
25. Allevato MAJ. Diseases mimicking onychomycosis. Clin Dermatol. 2010;28:164–77.
26. Bodman MA. Nail Dystrophies. Clin Podiatr Med Surg. 2004;21(4):663–87. viii
27. Zaiac MN, Daniel CR. Nails in systemic disease. Dermatol Ther. 2002;15(2):99–106.
28. Zaias N, Rebell G, Casal G, Appel J. The asymmetric gait toenail unit sign. Skinmed. 2012;10(4):213–7.
29. Zaias N, Rebell G, Escovar S. Asymmetric gait nail unit syndrome: the most common worldwide toenail abnormality and onychomycosis. Skinmed. 2014;12(4):217–23.
30. Vlahovic TC, Schleicher SM. "Nail disorders" in skin disease of the lower extremities: a photographic guide, HMP Communications, 2012.

Chapter 20
Onychomycosis: Procedures and Laser Treatment

Joseph Vella and Tracey C. Vlahovic

Introduction

Onychomycosis is a very common problem in the podiatric practice with a reported incidence of 3.22 % in the general population, ranging from 0.14 % in children to 11.93 % in at-risk populations such as dialysis patients [1]. Current therapies have mostly focused on oral antifungals and, more recently, topicals such as efinaconazole and tavaborole. It is true that the oral antifungals have repeatedly proven to be the most effective for toenail fungus, and the newer topical medications' increased efficacy is certainly encouraging. However, questions of their usefulness arise in patients in which these modalities are not affordable and/or plausible with concomitant medical issues. In these patients the question is: are there other modalities for treating nail fungal infections, whether it be distal lateral subungual onychomycosis or total dystrophic onychomycosis?

Recently that answer is in the affirmative with new modalities coming to market in the last few years. In the past, that answer involved surgical intervention with or without concomitant antifungal treatment. Various surgical methods were studied, including debridement, abrasion, avulsion, matrixectomy, and more. More recently, laser and light therapy has become an area of interest for researchers. This chapter will focus on these alternative therapies and discuss the latest research on their application and efficacy.

J. Vella, DPM
Impression Foot & Ankle, 201 W. Guadalupe Rd. Ste. 318, Gilbert, AZ 85233, USA
e-mail: drvella@impressionfoot.com

T.C. Vlahovic, DPM, FFPM RCPS (Glasg) (✉)
Department of Podiatric Medicine, Temple University School of Podiatric Medicine, 148 N 8th Street, Philadelphia, 19107 PA, USA
e-mail: traceyv@temple.edu

A. Tosti et al. (eds.), *Onychomycosis*, DOI 10.1007/978-3-319-44853-4_20

Procedures

Just as in bacterial infections in the diabetic foot, frequently surgical correction of a fungal infection is a viable option. Many already do this as a part of "routine nail care," which in the case of fungal nail infections can be considered a surgical removal. We may think we're simply trimming nails for patients' comfort, but we are also decreasing fungal burden as we remove those thick brittle distal nail portions, just as if we were removing the overlying bacterial contaminants in a wound debridement. In cases of very limited onychomycosis, such as a dermatophytoma within the nail or early distal lateral subungual onychomycosis, this may be enough to remove the entire fungal burden.

However, most of the time simple nail debridement is not enough to achieve complete fungal cure. Concomitant oral or topical antifungal therapy is usually required to completely eradicate the infection. Malay et al. in 2009 studied 55 patients with onychomycosis and compared "routine nail care" alone to nail debridement combined with topical antifungal therapy. Not surprisingly, none of the patients in the debridement-alone group achieved mycological cure while 76.74 % of those receiving combined therapy did [2]. Ameen et al. in 2014 also recommended adding antifungal therapy to debridement but weren't optimistic about its results even with avulsion due to a disappointing randomized controlled trial that came out about the same time [3].

Some have suggested that abrasion or nail drilling, rather than debridement, may be just as successful in eradication of the fungal infection. Tchernev et al. suggested surgical removal for resistant infections but recommended abrasion therapy or superficial scraping of the nail plate if possible [4]. On the contrary, Cursi et al. studied the efficacy of oral and topical antifungals combined with nail abrasion in 2013 [5]. They achieved only 32–36 % complete or partial cure in 25 patients after 12 months with 24 % recurrence even in those who did achieve cure. More studies need to be done in this regard.

Sometimes debridement even with antifungal therapy is not enough, though, and more drastic surgical procedures need to be done, such as avulsions or matrixectomies. Regarding avulsions, painful pressure due to a thick mycotic nail can easily be relieved with temporary removal of all or part of the nail, but concomitant topical or oral antifungal therapy is also required here or the result will be as short lived as the procedure [6]. Moreover, total nail avulsions should be avoided as they can lead to shrinkage of the nail bed, distal in-growing edge, and upward growth of the nail bed due to the loss of compressing forces of the nail plate [7]. Baran et al. in 1985 achieved total cure in 20 patients treated with partial nail avulsions combined with topical and systemic antifungal therapy; however, it took 6–18 months [8]. Lai et al. performed 33 nail avulsions in 32 patients more recently and achieved complete cure or almost complete cure in 88 % of patients, but these patients also received topical or systemic antifungal therapy [9].

When avulsions combined with antifungal therapy fail to provide relief, permanent matrixectomy should be considered. Despite popular belief, there are multiple ways of doing this. The most popular technique involves removal of all or part of a nail with the matrix attached and afterward applying a chemical such as 89 % phenol or 10 % sodium hydroxide to the matrix to prevent regrowth. Proponents of sodium hydroxide say that it has a higher success rate with less drainage and faster healing times [6]. In either case, a tourniquet should be used as any blood in the surgical field will dilute the chemical and decrease effectiveness. The chemical of choice is usually applied three to four times for 30 s each, after which it is rinsed with alcohol (in the case of sodium hydroxide, it is neutralized due to an acid-base reaction). Care should be taken to apply the chemical not only to the matrix but to the nail bed in order to get the ventral nail matrix and prevent regrowth.

Other methods of removing the nail exist but are much less frequently used. These include negative galvanic current, radio-wave electrical energy, carbon dioxide lasers, occlusive urea, and "cold-steel" procedures such as the Winograd, Frost, and Zadik nail procedures. Negative galvanic current produces heat and production of sodium hydroxide through electrolysis at the cathode that is applied to the matrix for 4–7 min. Frequent users of this technique report decreased post-op pain, inflammation, and drainage than chemical matrixectomy [6]. Radio-wave electrical energy was described by Hettinger et al. in 1991 and is applied directly to the matrix via a probe. It only takes 2–4 s and provides matrix destruction and hemostasis by an electrocautery effect. Users report less postoperative pain, swelling, and infection than other methods, but no data supports this. Obviously this method cannot be used in people with pacemakers [6]. So-called "cold-steel" procedures such as the Frost and Zadik are good for truly resistant cases, and they give the added benefit of access to exostoses needing removal.

Not all procedures are meant to remove nail, either; Gupta et al. in 2012 discussed innovative medical devices that utilized iontophoresis or ultrasound to increase the transport of medications across the nail plate [10]. Two devices in development used iontophoresis and electrical current to increase drug intake of the nail plate in cadaveric models, some 7–13 times higher penetration. They reference a trial with 38 subjects in which iontophoresis combined with topical terbinafine resulted in mycological cure in 84 % of patients in 12 weeks. Ultrasound also increased nail permeability in canine models by 1.5 times.

Laser Therapy

Laser therapy for fungal nails has been a hot topic in recent years. Many articles have claimed significant efficacy at fungal eradication with few to no side effects.

Recently multiple systematic reviews have analyzed the effectiveness of laser therapy in the treatment of onychomycosis, including Bristow in 2014 and Ledon et al. in the same year. Bristow's initial literature search brought up 268 articles, which was then narrowed down to 12 after excluding those which didn't meet inclusion criteria due to poor design, small sample size, and poor internal or external validity [11]. Even among the articles that did make the cut, Bristow had difficulty with analysis on a larger scale due to heterogeneity of study design and diagnostic methods. Additionally the follow-up period for most studies was 12–24 weeks even though it may actually take 24 months to fully evaluate the effectiveness on the nail fungus. No studies compared laser therapy with more traditional therapies like oral terbinafine or topical efinaconazole. Finally, only one study made no declaration of competing interests, making it hard to fully accept their findings without that nagging sense of bias in the back of the reader's mind.

Despite all this, there were some interesting trends and findings that may help those who are considering using laser therapy for onychomycosis and which device is the most effective. For example, the neodymium-doped yttrium aluminum garnet (Nd:YAG) laser seems to be the most frequently researched device, albeit with mixed results. Kalokasidis et al. in one of the larger studies treated 131 patients with microbiologically confirmed onychomycosis with a Q-switched Nd:YAG 1064/532 nm laser following nail reduction with a drill. After two treatments 30 days apart and using both wavelengths, they achieved a 95.4 % cure rate confirmed by microscopy and culture. Of note, only distal lateral subungual onychomycosis (DLSO) and superficial white onychomycosis (SWO) were studied, leaving readers to wonder whether this method would be as effective for more extensive infection such as total dystrophic onychomycosis (TDO) [11].

In another larger study, Zhang et al. used the 1064 nm Nd:YAG long pulse laser device to study 33 patients with 154 microscopically and culture-proven mycotic nails. Patients received either four or eight treatments at 1 week intervals, and results were tallied at 24 weeks. There was no significant difference in mycological cure rates between the two groups, but they did achieve 53 and 51 % mycological cure rates, respectively. They also reported a recurrence in ten nails within 2–4 months of treatment, suggesting that the laser only temporarily inhibited fungal growth in the nails [11].

On the other hand, Hollmig et al. studied the effectiveness of the 1064 nm Nd:YAG laser in 27 patients with culture or PAS stain confirmed onychomycosis. Patients received either no treatment or two laser treatments 2 weeks apart, with follow-up at both 3 months and 1 year. At 3 months, only 33 % of the laser group achieved negative culture as compared to 20 % in the control group with no statistically significant difference between the two groups. By 12 months there was no difference between the groups, suggesting again that laser may only have a temporary effect in onychomycosis [11].

One of the few studies not involving the Nd:YAG laser was done by Landsman et al. in 2010. In their randomized controlled trial, 36 patients with proven onychomycosis were randomly allocated to laser treatment using a continuous wave 870/930 nm laser or control sham device. Patients were treated at day 1, 14, 42, and 60. At 6 months, only two treated nails had completely or markedly improved (as well as two controls) with slight to moderate improvement in 18 treated nails and three control nails. The study was funded exclusively by a laser manufacturer with employees of the company listed as coauthors [11].

Another systematic review by Ledon et al. in 2014 studied a wider range of laser and light devices in the treatment of onychomycosis [12]. While still including studies about the Nd:YAG laser, they also analyzed studies of the carbon dioxide (CO_2) and dual wavelength 870/930 nm lasers, UV light therapy, and photodynamic therapy. They also made the observation that the FDA has approved laser systems for a "temporary increase in clear nail in patients with onychomycosis."

The CO_2 laser system was discussed first – appropriately, since it is the oldest laser therapy used for onychomycosis. A few early studies showed promising results with 66–75 % efficacy; however, these results were questionable due to confounding factors such as concurrent topical antifungal use, regular debulking, and failure to confirm clearance with culture. Moreover, new less invasive treatments have made this modality less desirable, and as such it is rarely used today [12].

UV light therapy was once a promising therapy for onychomycosis. It is known that UV light is extremely germicidal, which led researchers to investigate its use in onychomycosis. Indeed, Dai et al. studied in vitro susceptibility of *T. rubrum* to UVC light and achieved 100 % clearance at 144 J/cm^2 [12]. *T. rubrum* showed no resistance to this therapy, either. However, the mutagenic potential of UV light has limited its use and thus further studies of its efficacy.

Photodynamic therapy (PDT) consists of the combination of a photosensitizing agent (such as 5-aminolevulinic acid or 5-ALA) with irradiation by a specific wavelength of light. In vitro studies were promising, with one study by Donnelly et al. achieving 90 % reduction in viability with *C. albicans* and 79 % reduction in viability with *T. interdigitale*. In vivo studies were less promising though: one clinical trial evaluating PDT after chemical avulsion of the toenail reported a 43.3 % clinical and mycological cure rate after three sessions of 20 % 5-ALA for 3 h and at 12-month follow-up. Other small case studies had some success without the chemical nail avulsion. Some other photosensitizers, such as Sylsens B, have been shown to be effective in vitro, specifically against *T. rubrum*-infected human skin [12]. Ameen et al. also quoted a recent PDT study in which the researchers had obtained a 44.3 % cure rate at 12 months, which dropped to 36.6 % at 18 months [3]. They concluded that more studies need to be done, specifically on living human nails.

Dual wavelength 870/930 nm laser therapy has had limited success in the literature. Besides referencing the aforementioned article by Landsman et al., Ledon also found a small case study by Bornstein et al. with seven patients treated with four sessions of 870/930 nm laser therapy over the course of 60 days. In this small study, they observed a 100 % negative culture rate but only observed clear nail growth in four patients [12].

Conclusion

In summary, more research needs to be done on both alternative procedures as well as laser and light therapy in the treatment of onychomycosis. Although some of the research is promising and contains sound principles for treatment, varied study designs with small patient populations make it difficult to recommend these modalities. With the volume of research that has been done in recent years, it shouldn't be too long before we have solid evidence to guide us one way or the other. For now, pharmaceutical treatment with or without debridement and/or surgical removal remains the accepted standard of care.

Conflict of Interest The author has no conflicts of interest or financial disclosures.

References

1. Gupta AK, Daigle D, Foley KA. The prevalence of culture-confirmed toenail onychomycosis in at-risk patient populations. J Eur Acad Dermatol Venereol. 2015;29(6):1039–44.
2. Malay DS, Yi S, Borowsky P, et al. Efficacy of debridement alone versus debridement combined with topical antifungal nail lacquer for the treatment of pedal onychomycosis: a randomized, controlled trial. J Foot Ankle Surg. 2009;48:294–308.
3. Ameen M, Lear JT, Madan V, et al. British Association of Dermatologists' guidelines for the management of onychomycosis 2014. Br J Dermatol. 2014;171:937–58.
4. Tchernev G, Penev PK, Nenoff P, et al. Onychomycosis: modern diagnostic and treatment approaches. Wien Med Wochenschr. 2013;163(1–2):1–12.
5. Cursi IB, Silva RT, Succi IB, et al. Onychomycosis due to neoscytalidium treated with oral terbinafine, ciclopirox nail lacquer and nail abrasion: a pilot study of 25 patients. Mycopathologia. 2013;175:75–82.
6. McInnes BD, Dockery GL. Surgical treatment of mycotic toenails. JAPMA. 1997;87(12):557–64.
7. Grover C, Khurana A. An update on treatment of onychomycosis. Mycoses. 2012;55:541–51.
8. Baran R, Hay RJ. Partial surgical avulsion of the nail in onychomycosis. Clin Exp Dermatol. 1985;10:413–8.
9. Lai WY, Tang WY, Loo SK, et al. Clinical characteristics and treatment outcomes of patients undergoing nail avulsion surgery for dystrophic nails. Hong Kong Med J. 2011;17:127–31.
10. Gupta AK, Simpson FC. Medical devices for the treatment of onychomycosis. Dermatol Ther. 2012;25:574–81.
11. Bristow IR. The effectiveness of lasers in the treatment of onychomycosis: a systematic review. J Foot Ankle Res. 2014;7:34–43.
12. Ledon JA, Savas J, Franca K, et al. Laser and light therapy for onychomycosis: a systematic review. Lasers Med Sci. 2014;29:823–9.

Chapter 21
New Topical Antifungals

Tracey C. Vlahovic

Until recently, topical treatments for onychomycosis employed lacquer formulations (e.g., ciclopirox). These are organic solutions of film-forming polymers. Upon application to the surface of the nail, the solvent evaporates, leaving a water-resistant polymer film on the nail plate. This occlusive film acts as a drug reservoir that facilitates the release and penetration of the drug into and through the nail. One must then remove the film either mechanically or with organic solvents and apply fresh lacquer to replenish the drug reservoir [1, 2].

Efficacy in treating onychomycosis with ciclopirox lacquer reported complete cure rates range from 5.5 to 8.5 % [3]. Various authors have suggested that poor nail penetration is the main factor limiting the use of topical antifungal agents in the treatment of onychomycosis, directly relating to the nail plate's unique properties, its thickness and relatively compact structure, the physicochemical properties of the antifungal agent, and its formulation [4–10].

Chronic nail plate infection increases nail thickness [11, 12]. Other authors have noted that chronic nail plate infection creates a brittle nail unit, suggesting a more porous structure of the nail and erosion of the intracellular matrix that renders the tissue more permeable to topically applied agents especially when it is an aqueous-based vehicle formulation [13].

T.C. Vlahovic, DPM, FFPM RCPS (Glasg)
Department of Podiatric Medicine, Temple University School of Podiatric Medicine, 148 N 8th Street, Philadelphia, 19107 PA, USA
e-mail: traceyv@temple.edu

A. Tosti et al. (eds.), *Onychomycosis*, DOI 10.1007/978-3-319-44853-4_21

The Recently Approved Topical Antifungal Agents: Efinaconazole and Tavaborole

In 2014, two new topical solutions for onychomycosis were FDA approved: efinaconazole (Jublia, Valeant Pharmaceuticals) and tavaborole (Kerydin, PharmaDerm). The complete cure rates of tavaborole 5 % solution are 6.5–9.1 %, and the complete cure rates for efinaconazole 10 % solution are 15.2–17.8 % [14–16]. Both efinaconazole and tavaborole were studied in Phase 3 clinical trials where their protocols were not identical. In both studies, patients applied the topical antifungal or vehicle once daily for 48 weeks with a four-week follow-up; however, they vary in their percent nail involvement, age limit, and other criteria. Therefore, it is impossible to make a head-to-head comparison between both medications.

Elewski et al. assessed the efficacy, safety, and tolerability of efinaconazole in two double-blind, randomized, vehicle-controlled, multicenter studies in 1655 patients with mild to moderate onychomycosis (ranging between 20 and 50 % affected target toenail involvement) [16]. In addition to the aforementioned complete cure rates, researchers noted significantly greater mycologic cure rates (55.2 and 53.4 %) in efinaconazole-treated patients in comparison to the vehicle control.

Elewski and colleagues also studied tavaborole in two parallel designed studies of 1197 patients with mild to moderate onychomycosis (ranging between 20 and 60 % affected target toenail involvement) with slight differences in enrollment criteria [14, 15]. In the two studies, 26.1 and 27.5 percent of patients treated with tavaborole achieved a completely or almost clear nail at 52 weeks in comparison to 9.3 and 14.6 % in the vehicle groups. The study authors also noted that the rates of negative mycology in the tavaborole groups were 31.1 and 35.9 % in comparison to 7.2 and 12.2 % in the vehicle groups.

Lacquer-based topical therapies are applied primarily to the exterior nail plate, with drug reaching the infection site mostly through nail permeation [4, 5, 17]. Much has been written about topical onychomycosis treatments and the challenge of effective nail penetration following their application to the nail plate with the dorsal layer acting as the major barrier to penetration [18, 19]. Researchers have emphasized the need for the active ingredient to pass through the nail plate to reach the site of infection and have suggested a number of physicochemical factors (such as molecular size, hydrophilic or lipophilic nature of the agent, pH, ionic strength, and nature of the vehicle formulation) as important factors in influencing permeability [18]. Studies have reported variable nail permeability for all the available topical preparations available in the United States and work continues to find agents and formulation approaches to enhance nail penetration [20–23].

Efinaconazole is an alcohol-based solution that provides low surface tension and good wetting properties [24]. In a study of 11 patients with onychomycosis, Elewski et al. found that applying efinaconazole vehicle solution solely to the hyponychium spreads the topical into the subungual space between the nail plate and nail bed, reaching the site of infection [25]. Application to the hyponychium and ventral aspect of the nail plate may be important in patients wishing to continue to use nail polish [26]. Although nail polish does not appear to influence efinaconazole penetration into the nail, nail polish can become tacky with repeated application [27].

Tavaborole is also an alcohol-based solution that provides low surface tension but also boasts a low molecular weight-active ingredient that penetrates well through the human nail plate [16]. In a human cadaver nail study, tavaborole penetrated the nail plate 40 times greater than topical ciclopirox [28]. Up to four layers of nail polish does not seem to inhibit penetration of tavaborole [29]. In neither efinaconazole nor tavaborole has the impact of nail polish on efficacy been assessed, nor is it contraindicated.

As toenail growth progresses from proximal to distal, newly formed nail plate replaces diseased nail, a process that can take 12–18 months [29]. Clinical trial data suggest tavaborole and efinaconazole should be applied daily to the toenails for at least 48 weeks. Some patients may require treatment for considerably longer because of slow toenail growth, disease severity, or for other reasons. It is not known whether longer treatment regimens with tavaborole or efinaconazole would produce better efficacy results; however, higher cure rates following longer follow-up periods have been reported with other agents [30–32].

It is important that patients recognize that "cure" may not translate to a completely clear nail [33]. Poor adherence with any long-term chronic therapy is well documented [34]. A number of post hoc analyses with efinaconazole have been carried out to better identify prognostic factors for treatment success. Gender [35] and disease severity [36] were significant influencers of complete cure over the duration of the studies; female patients and those with milder disease may see results much quicker in clinical practice, whereas male patients and those with moderately severe disease may require a longer treatment course or combination therapy with oral antifungals. Although male patients are more difficult to treat, reasons are unclear. They tend to seek help for more advanced disease and suffer more nail trauma; toenails tend to be thicker. The reduced rate of growth and thickness of the nail may be factors in more severe disease, although it may be that these patients just require longer treatment courses.

Tinea pedis is an important causative factor for onychomycosis, and better results are seen when any coexisting tinea pedis is also treated [37]. In addition, managing tinea pedis is critical to minimizing disease recurrence.

Treatment Options for Current and Post-onychomycosis Toenail Onychodystrophy: Combination Therapy with Devices, Cosmetic, and Nutritional

During and after treatment of the underlying infection seen in onychomycosis, the nail plate may not regain its original healthy appearance. Clinicians should consider other therapies and devices to use in combination with an antifungal therapy and/or use post topical antifungal therapy that will adhere to the nail plate, provide mechanical support, and be easy to use.

There are two medical devices available for the treatment of onychodystrophy: Genadur™ (hydroxypropyl chitosan, Medimetriks) and Nuvail™ (poly-ureaurethane, 16 %, Cipher). These are nondrug lacquers applied topically to the nail at bedtime. Genadur is indicated to "protect damaged nails from the effects of moisture, friction, or shear" in order to relieve the symptoms of nail dystrophy [38]. It is a hydrosoluble compound that should be applied after nail washing and drying. Studies on psoriatic nails have shown that it has an improvement in nail fragility, a reduction in splitting, and a 63 % reduction in onycholysis [39].

Nuvail is a waterproof and flexible film that forms to the nail contour to provide protection from direct abrasion and provides optimal moisture balance to protect the nail from the effects of moisture [40]. Nasir et al. followed 53 patients with nail dystrophy who used Nuvail nightly [41]. Clinical assessment, which evaluated color, onycholysis, and subungual hyperkeratosis, resulted in a 60 % improvement after 6 months of use.

In addition, if cosmesis is a concern for the patient, Keryflex™ nail resin may be applied to camouflage and protect the nail unit. A podiatric office-based therapy, Keryflex™ (Podiatree Company), has been used to cover nail fungus and various other nail dystrophies whether the patient is being systemically treated for the underlying condition or not. Among its many uses, it has been applied following the use of the laser for onychomycosis and in covering a nail that has become dystrophic following surgery for paronychia. It is a flexible nail resin that is not suitable for fingernails, as it moves with the foot and takes some impact of external forces, making it suitable for use in athletes and dancers who regularly traumatize the toenails.

Biotin, an oral option for brittle nails, benefits dystrophic nails approximately 2–3 months after starting the supplement [42]. Although there is no protocol on optimal duration of use, biotin supplementation should continue as long as there is clinical improvement.

Conclusion

Onychomycosis will remain a common nail disease that should be treated effectively and early to prevent progression into a more severe, debilitating, and painful condition. In addition, prevalence will likely continue to increase as the population ages, and more patients seek treatment due to resurgence of media interest. Product development will focus on physicochemical properties suited to treating onychomycosis and advances in formulation research to ensure sufficient product reaches the site of infection in the nail bed. It is likely that other routes to the infection (not just permeability through the nail plate) will become important.

One area of research that is likely in the future is the potential of other penetration routes for topical therapy. The benefits of subungual delivery are clear, and a dual approach of transungual delivery and application under the hyponychium could provide greater efficacy. Subungual delivery may also be an important consideration for those patients who either want to continue to use nail polish or wish to start using nail polish once they see improvement in the toenail.

With more new topical products entering the market, we are likely to see increased patient awareness and expectation. Education of our patients in terms of disease management, how long it takes for the nail to become normal, and what they can do to prevent disease spreading or reinfection will be critical.

References

1. Murdan S. The nail: anatomy, physiology, diseases and treatment. In: Murthy SN, Maibach HI, editors. Topical nail products and ungual drug delivery. Boca Raton: Taylor and Francis Group, CRC Press; 2013. p. 1–36.
2. Sparavigna A, Setaro M, Frisenda L. Physical and microbiological properties of a new nail protective medical device. J Plastic Dermatol. 2008;4(1):5–12.
3. Gupta AK, Joseph WS. Ciclopirox 8 % nail lacquer in the treatment of onychomycosis of the toenails in the United States. J Am Podiatr Med Assoc. 2000;90(10):495–501.
4. Baran R, Kaoukhov A. Topical antifungal drugs for the treatment of onychomycosis: an overview of current strategies for monotherapy and combination therapy. J Eur Acad Dermatol Venereol. 2005;19(1):21–9.
5. Lecha M, Effendy I, de Chauvin M F, Di Chiacchio N, Baran R. Treatment options—development of consensus guidelines. J Eur Acad Dermatol Venereol. 2005;19(Suppl 1):25–33.
6. Murdan S. Drug delivery to the nail following topical application. Int J Pharm. 2002;236(1–2):1–26.
7. Baker SJ, Hui X, Maibach HI. Progress on new therapeutics for fungal nail infections. Annu Rep Med Chem. 2005;40:323–34.
8. Mertin D, Lippold BC. In-vitro permeability of the human nail and of a keratin membrane from bovine hooves: influence of the partition coefficient octanol/water and the water solubility of drugs on their permeability and maximum flux. J Pharm Pharmacol. 1997;49(1):30–4.
9. Kobayashi Y, Komatsu T, Sumi M, Numajiri S, et al. In vitro permeation of several drugs through the human nail plate: relationship between physicochemical properties and nail permeability of drugs. Eur J Pharm Sci. 2004;21(4):471–7.
10. Tatsumi Y, Yokoo M, Senda H, Kakehi K. Therapeutic efficacy of topically applied KP-103 against experimental tinea unguium in guinea pigs in comparison with amorolfine and terbinafine. Antimicrob Agents Chemother. 2002;46(12):3797–801.
11. Baraldi A, Jones SA, Guesne S, et al. Human nail plate modifications induced by onychomycosis: implications for topical therapy. Pharm Res. 2015;32(5):1626–33.
12. Tosti A, Daniel R, Piraccini BM, Iorizzo M. Color atlas of nails. Berlin: Springer; 2010. p. 15–22.
13. Hamilton JB, Terada H, Mestler GE. Studies of growth throughout the lifespan in Japanese: growth and size of nails and their relationship to age, sex, heredity, and other factors. J Gerontol. 1955;10(4):401–15.
14. Elewski BE, Rich P, Wiltz H, et al. Effectiveness and safety of tavaborole, a novel boron-based molecule for the treatment of onychomycosis: results from two phase 3 studies. Poster presented at Winter Clinical Meeting. Waimea: Hawaii; 2014.
15. Elewski BE, Aly R, Baldwin SL, et al. Efficacy and safety of tavaborole topical solution, 5 %, a novel boron-based antifungal agent, for the treatment of onychomycosis: results from 2 randomized phase-III studies. J Am Acad Dermatol. 2015;73:62–9. doi:10.1016/j.jaad.2015.04.010.

16. Elewski BE, Rich P, Pollak R, et al. Efinaconazole 10 % solution in the treatment of toenail onychomycosis: two phase III multicenter, randomized, double-blind studies. J Am Acad Dermatol. 2013;68(4):600–8.
17. Singh G, Haneef NS, Uday A. Nail changes and disorders among the elderly. Indian J Dermatol Venereol Leprol. 2005;71(6):386–92.
18. Thatai P, Sapra B. Transungual delivery: deliberations and creeds. Int J Cosmet Sci. 2014;36(5):398–411.
19. Kobayashi Y, Miyamoto M, Sugibayashi K, et al. Drug permeation through the three layers of the human nail plate. J Pharm Pharmacol. 1999;51(3):271–8.
20. Monti D, Tampucci S, Chetoni P, et al. Ciclopirox vs amorolfine: in vitro penetration through human health nails of commercial nail lacquers. J Drugs Dermatol. 2014;13(2):143–7.
21. Monti D, Saccomani L, Chetoni P, et al. Validation of bovine hoof slices as a model for infected human toenails: in vitro ciclopirox transungual permeation. Br J Dermatol. 2011;165(1):99–105.
22. Hui X, Baker SJ, Wester RC, et al. In vitro penetration of a novel oxaborole antifungal (AN 2690) into the human nail plate. J Pharm Sci. 2007;96(10):2622–31.
23. Sakamoto M, Sugimoto N, Kawabata H, et al. Transungual delivery of efinaconazole: its deposition in the nail of onychomycosis patients and in vivo fungicidal activity in the human nails. J Drugs Dermatol. 2014;13(11):1338–92.
24. Bhatt V, Pillai R. Efinaconazole topical solution, 10 %: formulation development program of a new topical treatment of toenail onychomycosis. J Pharm Sci. 2015;104:2177–82. doi:10.1002/jps.24459.
25. Elewski BE, Pollak RA, Pillai R, et al. Access of efinaconazole topical solution 10 % to the infection site by spreading through the subungual space. J Drugs Dermatol. 2014;13(11):1394–8.
26. Elewski BE, Pollak RA, Pillai R, et al. Access of efinaconazole topical solution, 10 %, to the infection site by spreading through the subungual space. J Drugs Dermatol. 2014;13:1394–8.
27. Zeichner JA, Stein Gold L, Korotzer A. Penetration of (14C)-efinaconazole solution does not appear to be influenced by Nail Polish. J Clin Aesthet Dermatol. 2014;7(9):45–8.
28. Elewski BE, Tosti A. Tavaborole for the treatment of onychomycosis. Expert Opin Pharmacother. 2014;15(10):1439–48.
29. Vlahovic T, Merchant T, Chanda S, et al. In vitro nail penetration of tavaborole topical solution, 5 % through nail polish on ex vivo human fingernails. J Drugs Dermatol. 2015;14(7):675–8.
30. Del Rosso JQ. Advances in the treatment of superficial fungal infections: focus on onychomycosis and dry tinea pedis. J Am Osteopath Assoc. 1997;97:339–46.
31. Sigurgeirsson B, Billstein S, Rantanen T, et al. L.I.ON. Study: efficacy and tolerability of continuous terbinafine compared to intermittent itraconazole in the treatment of toenail onychomycosis. Br J Dermatol. 1999;141(Supp 56):5–14.
32. Baran R, Tosti A, Hartmane I, et al. An innovative water-soluble biopolymer improves efficacy of ciclopirox nail lacquer in the management of onychomycosis. J Eur Acad Dermatol Venereol. 2009;23:773–81.
33. Baran R, Sigurgeirsson B, de Berker D, et al. A multicenter, randomized, controlled study of the efficacy, safety and cost-effectiveness of a combination therapy with amorolfine nail lacquer and oral terbinafine compared with oral terbinafine alone for the treatment of onychomycosis. Br J Dermatol. 2007;157(1):149–57.
34. Hay RJ. The future of onychomycosis therapy may involve a combination of approaches. Br J Dermatol. 2001;145:3–8.
35. Rosen T. Evaluation of gender as a clinically relevant outcome variable in the treatment of onychomycosis with efinaconazole topical solution 10 %. Cutis. 2015;96(3):197–201.
36. Rodriguez DA. Efinaconazole topical solution, 10 % for the treatment of mild and moderate toenail onychomycosis. J Clin Aesthet Dermatol. 2015;8(6):24–9.
37. Markinson B, Caldwell B. Efinaconazole topical solution, 10 %: efficacy in onychomycosis patients with co-existing tinea pedis. J Am Podiatr Med Assoc. 2015;105(5):407–11.

38. Genadur PI. Medimetriks. http://medimetriks.com/PIs/Genadur_PI.pdf.
39. Cantoresi F, Sorgi P, Arcese A, et al. Improvement of psoriatic onychodystrophy by a water-soluble nail lacquer. J Eur Acad Dermatol Venereol. 2009 Jul;23(7):832–4.
40. Nuvail PI. Innocutis. http://innocutis.com/wp-content/uploads/2012/06/nuvail-pi_0612.pdf.
41. Nasir A, Goldstein B, van Cleff M, Swick L. Clinical evaluation of safety and efficacy of a new topical treatment for onychomycosis. J Drugs Dermatol. 2011;10(10):1186–91.
42. Scheinfeld N, Dahdah MJ, Scher R. Vitamins and minerals: their role in nail health and disease. J Drugs Dermatol. 2007;6(8):782–7.

Chapter 22
New Topical and Systemic Antifungals

Gabriela Moreno-Coutiño and Roberto Arenas

Key Features

1. Still in search for the ideal onychomycosis treatment
2. New topical treatments predominate over systemic ones
3. Many studies are focused on nail plate permeability
4. Risk factors must be considered to determine which is the best therapy for each case
5. Refractory cases are usually secondary to non-dermatophytes molds.

Introduction

Onychomycosis is a chronic and progressive fungal infection of the nail plate that causes destruction and deformity of the normal structures with the consequent discomfort and psychological stress for which patients pursue the cure.

The history of antifungal drugs (Table 22.1) began in the 1950s with the development of amphotericin B, a polyene of the same family as nystatin and pimaricin. Griseofulvin the first anti-dermatophyte oral drug was FDA approved almost in 1960. Afterward came 5-fluorocytosine and the azoles in the 1970s with the newest one approved by the FDA in 2015, isavuconazonium sulfate [1, 2].

Allylamines, terbinafine and naftifine, appeared in the 1990s and amorolfine years later. Echinocandins, as anidulafungin, caspofungin, and micafungin, were initially used around 1980.

G. Moreno-Coutiño, MD • R. Arenas, MD (✉)
Mycology Section, Dr. Manuel Gea González General Hospital, México, DF, México
e-mail: gmorenocoutino@gmail.com; rarenas98@hotmail.com

A. Tosti et al. (eds.), *Onychomycosis*, DOI 10.1007/978-3-319-44853-4_22

Table 22.1 Main antimycotic groups

Polyenes
Azoles
Allylamines
B-Glucan synthase inhibitors (echinocandins)
Pyrimidine analogues
Mitotic inhibitors
Aminoacyl-tRNA synthetase inhibitors
Others

Some have fungistatic, fungicide, or mixed action. Many of them are broad-spectrum drugs that can be used in superficial and/or systemic fungal infections. However, although the list of antimycotics is long and continues to grow, the development of new antifungal agents is rather slow if compared to the development of new antibiotics, despite the growing number of systemic mycosis. The main reason is the similitudes shared by human and fungal cells which are eukaryotes and thus can be more toxic to humans in a parallel manner. They also cause drug interactions and hepatic or renal toxicity more frequently than antibiotics. For this reason, the major developments on new systemic drugs are almost exclusively reserved for systemic life-threatening mycoses [3].

So, even if onychomycosis is the most common nail disease and it's prevalence increases with age and with the growing immunosuppressed population, the development of novel drugs required for its cure is not focused on being systemic but rather a topical and extremely effective option that, to this moment, we are lacking. Despite adequate treatment, more than 20 % of the onychomycosis that receive oral treatment don't resolve, even when combined with an adjuvant topical option [4, 5].

Diffusion Treatments

Onychomycosis is cosmopolite and affects around 8 % of the population with its prevalence and causal agents more or less similar worldwide.

Commonly dermatophytes are responsible for the infection, but yeasts and non-dermatophyte molds (NDM) can be isolated. The incidence increases with age and is associated to other diseases such as peripheral vascular insufficiency, diabetes, and any other form of immunosuppression [6].

The prevalence in patients older than 60 years of age is 20 % but dramatically increases to 50 % 10 years later. This can be added to the risk in diabetic patients that is 1.9–2.8 times higher when compared to nondiabetics. In HIV-positive patients, the prevalence ranges from 15 to 40 % [7].

All therapeutic options, systemic or topical, new or old, still pose the disadvantage of prolonged administration. To this moment the standard treatment is oral terbinafine or itraconazole with cure rates of 76 % for the former and 63 % for the latter, and fluconazole has a cure rate of only 48 % [7, 8].

These three antifungals present very similar results among adults and children [9]. However, as the elderly are the most affected age group, drug interactions and liver toxicity frequently discourage systemic administration of antimycotics, so topical agents are preferred. Despite these innovations, there still is the need for a superior option because the cure rate is still very poor [10, 11].

A study analyzed the cases of initially negative KOH results for onychomycosis and concluded that up to 94 % of the tests reported as negative, after more thorough examinations turned out to be positive, so the authors conclude that the systemic antifungal treatment should be indicated on a clinical diagnosis. We personally disagree, because these depend on two important factors which are the experience and skills of the person performing the KOH mount and the clinical ability for onychomycosis diagnosis of the physician [12]. We must also consider what Feuilhade de Chauvin mentions that the fungal species need to be identified for the correct antifungal election, as yeasts and NDM can also cause onychomycosis, despite the fact that dermatophytes are the most common etiological agents [13].

The American Academy of Dermatology reinforced the recommendation for confirmatory testing of onychomycosis before initiating systemic treatment with the intention to reduce unnecessary side effects and economic burden; although they also recognize that overall confirmatory testing is more expensive than treating all suspected cases and that the potentially harmful side effects secondary to oral treatment (usually terbinafine or itraconazole) are extremely infrequent [14].

So, if we are on a clinical setting, we will most commonly seek confirmatory testing, but if our aim is optimization of resources, we most likely won't solicit them and both options are ethically supported.

Treatment

Systemic

About the first line of oral treatment for onychomycosis, there is no news. Terbinafine and itraconazole are still the ones we must choose from, the former considered the gold standard [15–18].

However, what may be an improvement is the sequential therapy, which is the combination of two oral antifungals that act in different pathways of ergosterol metabolism, with the intention to reduce duration of treatment. For this, patients are given two pulses of itraconazole and, afterward, one or two of terbinafine [19–21].

Fluconazole is a hydro and keratinophilic azole with actions similar to those of itraconazole, dependent on the CYP450 system is used as weekly dosage treatment for onychomycosis during 6–9 months, and is not FDA approved for this purpose [22] but sometimes selected by its covenient posology and broad spectrum.

As *Candida* sp. and non-dermatophyte molds (NDM) can also cause onychomycosis, these fungi are frequently encountered as unresponsive to the first line of treatment. Voriconazole, an azole usually reserved for severe systemic fungal infections, has been successful in refractory NDM onychomycosis (*Scytalidium dimidiatum*). One report mentions excellent results in a patient with total onychodystrophy of a fingernail and tinea in both hands and feet. She was treated during 3 months monitoring the drug plasma levels [23–25].

Posaconazole has proven in vitro to have a potent antifungal activity against dermatophytes.

A phase 2 clinical trial of posaconazole in the treatment of onychomycosis receiving 100, 200, or 400 mg once a day during 24 weeks or 400 mg once a day for 12 weeks showed that the diffusion of the drug to the nail plate is similar to other antifungals such as itraconazole or terbinafine, and the levels in the nail plate remain high after treatment is stopped, which suggests that it accumulates in the nail matrix [17, 26].

Posaconazole weekly dosages during a month were indicated to an HIV-positive patient with proximal white onychomycosis caused by *Fusarium falciforme* and resistant to itraconazole and terbinafine. With this regimen, mycological and clinical cure was obtained and sustained for at least 16 months [27].

Albaconazole is a broad-spectrum antifungal drug with activity against dermatophytes and NDM in vitro and in animal models. It has been studied in phase I and II for superficial dermatophytosis. Phase III is still pending [28].

Pramiconazole is another systemic azole commercialized in the late 2000s. This drug is one of the few developed specifically for superficial mycosis such as tinea versicolor, corporis, pedis, cruris, and onychomycosis. Clinical trials, phases I and II, were successfully reported with similar or superior antifungal activity as ketoconazole and itraconazole. A good absorption and a long half-life, so much that a daily dosage was sufficient, have been reported. It has been proved growth reduction in *Candida albicans*, *Malassezia globosa, Microsporum canis*, *Trichophyton mentagrophytes*, and *Trichophyton rubrum*. However, after these promising results, the laboratory was sold to another pharmaceutical company and the studies were put on hold [29].

This antimycotic was then used as an oral treatment for seborrheic dermatitis and vulvovaginitis as a phase IIa trial with promising results for yeast infections. However, no further studies with oral therapy have been conducted regarding dermatophyte infections [30, 31]. In vitro studies found that pramiconazole has activity against dermatophytes and yeasts with application of this topical antifungal, comparable with the results obtained with oral administration of itraconazole, miconazole, and terbinafine [32].

Although this is not directly related to antifungal drugs, it has been documented that patients living with HIV and onychomycosis can improve or even cure after the initiation of the combined antiretroviral therapy. These results may be multifactorial and further studies need to be conducted; however, this kind of recovery is not seen in the setting of other diseases that condition immunosuppression under the required specific treatment [33].

Topical

Ciclopirox hydro-lacquer is based on water soluble biopolymer technology which is supposed to be an improvement with previous lacquers, and still studies are being performed with terbinafine nail solution [19].

Naftifine hydrochloride 1 % in gel has proven usefulness in treating fingernail onychomycosis, of the distal subungual variety, with reasonable results and few side effects [34].

Several studies have been recently published about topical efinaconazole in 10 % solution which has been in the market for a couple of years. This azole derivate has been studied for its efficacy, safety, and tolerability as treatment for mild to moderate onychomycosis with results superior to the vehicle which contains alcohol, lipophilic esters, and cyclomethicone. After 52 weeks of treatment 18.5 % of patients showed complete cure, compared to 4.7 % of the control group. Mycologic cure was registered in 56.3 % and complete or partial cure in 2.7 %, and another interesting data obtained is that the mean unaffected new nail growth was higher with efinaconazole when compared to patients that received only the vehicle [35, 36].

Efinaconazole has been tested for toxicity, which is positive during gestation of rats, but not of rabbits. Is not teratogenic either to rats or rabbits [37–39].

In conclusion of all the reports published about 10 % topical efinaconazole, authors agree that it is a safe and effective option, particularly for mild onychomycosis and that, like any other previously tried topical treatment, can work as adjuvant in patients that are receiving systemic therapy. And although by its administration route, no life-threatening adverse reactions are expected, contact dermatitis has been reported [40, 41].

Tavaborole topical solution 5 % is a new treatment option. It is a broad-spectrum antifungal from the benzoxaboroles group that has been tested in phase III trials for efficacy and safety of onychomycosis both in adult and geriatric patients [42, 43]. It has a low molecular weight compared to other topical antifungals, which may enhance nail plate penetration although it showed a low mycological cure rate of 30–36 % [44, 45].

Outlook: Future Developments

The nail unit inherently requires a thick and resistant structure in order to resist environmental and occupational hazards and must be taken into account for the new treatment options.

A downside to topical treatments is the extremely long time the drug needs to be applied (e.g., 12 months for toenails), so an alternative to improve topical medications is to enhance drug penetration through the nail plate. A study on nail plate permeation to topical antifungal drugs found that onychomycosis infection changes nail permeability, opening the nail pores, and, thus, facilitates the passage of hydrophilic molecules, while the hydrophobic molecules did not show any improvement. The authors suggest that the change induced by the nail infection should be used as an advantage, and a small molecular weight hydrophilic antifungal agent with low levels of keratin binding could be of benefit [46, 47].

Other strategies are being developed in order to improve topical drugs penetration. These techniques include iontophoresis, nail abrasion, microporation, laser nail ablation, and laser therapy, among others [19].

The drug ME1111 [2-(3,5-dimethyl-1H-pyrazol-1-yl)-5-methylphenol is being developed as a new drug against dermatophytes, but still is under study [10].

Ravuconazole is a broad-spectrum azole that so far has been tried only for systemic mycoses and Chagas disease [48].

Luliconazole is a topical azole that has undergone phase I and IIa trials and case studies as topical treatment for onychomycosis as 10 % solution which reached steady plasma levels of the drug. It has also been tested in vitro against *Trichophyton rubrum* and *Trichophyton mentagrophytes*. The authors reached the conclusion that this drug has potent fungicidal activity when compared to the other topical azoles and promises good results as a therapeutic option in the near future. It has shown to be more potent than lanoconazole among other antifungals [49–52].

Miltefosine, which is an alkyphospholipid used to treat leishmaniasis and cutaneous breast metastasis, has now been proved to have potent in vitro activity against biofilms of *Fusarium oxysporum* and *Candida albicans*. So, probably in the near future, more studies will be performed with this drug that promises good results as topical treatment for non-dermatophyte onychomycosis [53].

Combination therapy of oral/oral, oral/topical, oral/laser, and topical/laser is still being tried in numerous studies with variable but modest results [54].

Apparently, the oral treatment options will stay the same, at least for some time. In vitro antifungal susceptibility studies mention terbinafine as the most potent antifungal against dermatophytes, followed by itraconazole and fluconazole [55].

And of course, we must not forget that prevention of risk factors will always play an important role in patients' lives [7].

Summary for the Clinician

Since onychomycosis is very common and the ideal treatment does not exist, many therapeutic approaches are available with variable results. Although it is a disadvantage, we can make the most of it by having countless treatments that can adapt to the social and medical needs of each of our patients, always taking into consideration the general health status, socioeconomic capacity, age, and possible drug interactions.

Clinical Pearls

When possible, onychomycosis diagnosis should be confirmed by KOH mount and culture.

Even after successful mycological cure, nail may persist dystrophic since clinical cure takes longer.

New treatments will continue under investigation to improve outcome.

References

1. Dixon DM, Walsh TJ. Chapter 76: Antifungal agents. In: Baron S, editor. Medical microbiology. 4th ed. Galveston: Univ of Texas Merdical Branch; 1996.
2. Azanza JR, García-Quetglas E, Sádaba B. Farmacología de los azoles. Rev Iberoam Micol. 2007;24:223–7.
3. Lewis RE. Current concepts in antifungal pharmacology. Mayo Clin Proc. 2011;86:805–17.
4. Baran R, Rigopoulos D. Nail therapies. Chapter 4B. London: Informa Healthcare; 2010. p. 17–29.
5. Barber K, Barber J. Onychomycosis: therapy directed by morphology and mycology. Skin Therapy Lett. 2009;14:1–2.
6. Ribeiro CS, Zaitz C, Framil VM, Ottoboni TS, Tonoli MS, Ribeiro RP. Descriptive study of onychomycosis in a hospital in Sao Paulo. Braz J Microbiol. 2015;46:485–92.
7. Westerberg DP, Voyack MJ. Onychomycosis: current trends in diagnosis and treatment. Am Fam Physician. 2013;88:762–70.
8. Coelho de Sá D, Bottolamas AP, Tosti A. Oral therapy for onychomycosis: an evidence based review. Am J Clin Dermatol. 2014;15:17–36.
9. Gupta AK, Paquet M. Systemic antifungals to treat onychomycosis in children: a systematic review. Pediatr Dermatol. 2013;30:294–302.
10. Takahata S, Kubota N, Takei-Masuda N, Yamada T, Maeda M, Mahdi Alshahni M, Abe S, Tabata Y, Maebashi K. Mechanism of action of ME1111, a novel antifungal agent for topical treatment of onychomycosis. Antimicrob Agents Chemother. 2016;60:873–80.
11. Vilaverde Schmitt J, Bombonatto G, Trierweiler SM, Buosi Fabri A. General aspects of drug interactions with systemic antifungals in a retrospective study sample. An Bras Dermatol. 2013;88:476–9.
12. Amichai B, Davidovici B, Trau H, Lyakhovitsky A, Grunwaldt MH, Shemer A. A rationale for systemic treatment in onychomycosis with negative results on fungal examination. Clin Exp Dermatol. 2011;36:724–7.
13. Feuilhade de Chauvin M. Traitement des onychomycoses. J Mycologie Medicale. 2014;24: 296–302.
14. Mikailov A, Cohen J, Joyce C, Mostaghimi A. Cost-effectiveness of confirmatory testing before treatment of onychomycosis. JAMA Dermatol. 2016;152:276–81.
15. Yin Z, Xu J, Luo D. A meta-analysis comparing long-term recurrences of toenail onychomycosis after successful treatment with terbinafine versus itraconazole. J Dermatol Treat. 2012;23:449–52.
16. Yadav P, Singal A, Pandhi D, Das S. Comparative efficacy of continuous and pulse dose terbinafine regimes inn toenail dermatophytosis: a randomized double-blind trial. Indian J Dermatol Venereol Leprol. 2015;81:363–9.
17. Gupta AK, Simpson FC. New pharmacotherapy for the treatment of onychomycosis: an update. Expert Opin Pharmacother. 2015;16:227–36.
18. Eldrige ML, Chambers CJ, Sharon VR, Thompson III GR. Fungal infections of the skin and nail: new treatment options. Expert Rev Anti Infect Ther. 2014;12:1389–405.
19. Singal A, Khanna D. Onychomycosis: diagnosis and management. Indian J Dermatol Venereol Leprol. 2011;77:659–72.
20. Bueno JG, Martinez C, Zapata B, Sanclemente G, Gallego M, Mesa AC. In vitro activity of fluconazole, itraconazole, voriconazole and terbinafine against fungi causing onychomycosis. Clin Exp Dermatol. 2009;35:658–63.
21. Ataides FS, Chaul MH, El Essal FE, Costa CR, Souza LKH, Fernandes OFL, Silva MRR. Antifungal susceptibility patterns of yeasts and filamentous fungi isolated from nail infection. J Eur Acad Dermatol Venereol. 2012;26:1479–85.
22. Welsh O, Vera-Cabrera L, Welsh E. Onychomycosis. Clin Dermatol. 2010;28:151–9.
23. Spriet I, Lambrecht C, Lagrou K, Verhamme B. Successful eradication of Scytalidium dimidiatum-induced ungula and cutaneous infection with voriconazole. Eur J Dermatol. 2012; 22:197–9.

24. Baudraz-Rosselet F, Ruffieux C, Lurati M, Bontems O, Monod M. Onychomycosis insensitive to systemic terbinafine and azole treatments reveals non dermatophyte moulds as infectious agents. Dermatol. 2010;220:164–8.
25. Badali H, Fakhim H, Zarei F, Nabili M, Vaezi A, Poorzad N, Dolatabadi S, Mirhendi H. In vitro activities of five antifungal drugs against opportunistic agents of Aspergillus nigri complex. Mycopathologia. 2015; doi:10.1007/s11046-015-9968-0.
26. Krishna G, Ma L, Martinho M, Prasad P, Wahl J, Tavakkol A. Determination of posaconazole levels in toenails of adults with onychomycosis following oral treatment with four regimens of posaconazole for 12 or 24 weeks. Antimicrob Agents Chemother. 2011;55:4424–6.
27. Al-Hatmi AMS, Bonifaz A, Calderón L, Curfs-Breuker I, Meis JF, van Diepeningen AD. Proximal subungual onychomycosis caused by Fusarium falciforme successfully cured with posaconazole. Br J Dermatol. 2015;173:253–5.
28. Guillon R, Pagniez F, Picot C, Hédou D, Tonnerre A, Chosson E, Duflos M, Besson T, Logé C, Le Pape P. Discovery of a novel broad-spectrum antifungal agent derived from albaconazole. ACS Med Chem Lett. 2013;4:288–92.
29. Geria AN, Scheinfeld NS. Pramiconazole, a triazole compound for the treatment of fungal infections. J Drugs Dermatol. 2008;11:661–70.
30. Donders G, Ausma J, Wouters L, Cauwenbergh G, Borgers M, Janssens D. Efficacy of a single oral dose of 200 mg pramiconazole in vulvovaginal yeast infections: an exploratory phase IIa trial. Acta Derm Venereol. 2008;88:462–6.
31. Gupta AK, Richardson M, Paquet M. Systematic review of oral treatments for seborrheic dermatitis. J Eur Acad Dermatol Venereol. 2014;28:16–26.
32. de Wit K, Paulussen C, Matheeussen A, van Rossem K, Cos P, Maes L. In vitro profiling of pramiconazole and in vivo evaluation in Microsporum canis dermatitis and *Candida albicans* vaginitis laboratory models. Antimicrob Agents Chemother. 2010;54:4927–9.
33. Ruíz-López P, Moreno-Coutiño G, Fernández-Martínez R, Espinoza-Hernández J, Rodríguez-Zulueta P, Reyes-Terán G. Evaluation of improvement of onychomycosis in HIV-infected patients after initiation of combined antiretroviral therapy without antifungal treatment. Mycoses. 2015;58:516–21.
34. Meyerson MS, Scher RK, Hochman LG, Cohen JL, Pappert AS, Holwell JE. Cutis. 1993;51:205–7.
35. Tosti A, Elewski BE. Treatment of onychomycosis with efinaconazole 10 % topical solution and quality of life. J Clin Aesthet Dermatol. 2014;7:25–306.
36. LaSenna CE, Tosti A. Patient considerations in the management of toe onychomycosis: role of efinaconazole. Patient Prefer Adherence. 2015;5:887–91.
37. Glynn M, Jo W, Minowa K, Sanada H, Nejishima H, Matsuuchi H, Okamura H, Pillai R, Mutter L. Efinaconazole: developmental and reproductive toxicity potential of a novel antifungal azole. Reprod Toxicol. 2015;52:18–25.
38. Rodriguez DA. Efinaconazole topical solution, 10 %, for the treatment of mild and moderate toenail onychomycosis. J Clin Aesthet Dermatol. 2015;8:24–9.
39. Lipner SR, Scher RK. Efinaconazole in the treatment of onychomycosis. Infect Drug Resist. 2015;8:163–72.
40. Gupta AK, Cernea M. How effective is efinaconazole in the management of onychomycosis? Expert Opin Pharmacother. 2016;17:611–8.
41. Hirohata A, Hanafusa T, Mabuchi-Kiyohara E, Ikegami R. Contact dermatitis caused by efinaconazole solution for treatment of onychomycosis. Contact Dermatitis. 2015;73:182–93.
42. Elewski BE, Tosti A. Tavaborole for the treatment of onychomycosis. Expert Opin Pharmacother. 2014;15:1439–48. Elewski BE, Aly R, Baldwin SL, González-Soto RF, Rich P, Weisfeld M, Wiltz H, Zane LT, Pollak R. Efficacy and safety of tavaborole topical solution, 5 %, a novel boron-based antifungal agent, for the treatment of toenail onychomycosis: results from 2 randomized phase III studies. J Am Acad Dermatol. 2015;73:62–9.
43. Del Rosso JQ. The role of topical antifungal therapy for onychomycosis and the emergence of newer agents. JN Clin Aesthet Dermatol. 2014;7:10–8.

44. Jinna S, Finch J. Spotlight on tavaborole for the treatment of onychomycosis. Drug Des Devel Ther. 2015;9:6185–90.
45. Sharma N, Sharma D. An upcoming drug for onychomycosis: tavaborole. J Pharm Pharmacol. 2015;6:236–9.
46. McAuley WJ, Jones SA, Traynor MJ, Guesné S, Murdan S, Brown MB. An investigation of how fungal infection influences drug penetration through onychomycosis patient's nail plates. Eur J Pharm Biopharm. 2016. doi. http://dx.doi.org/10.1016/j.ejpb.2016.03.008.
47. Elewski BE, Tosti A. Risk factors and comorbidities for onychomycosis. Implications for treatment with topical therapy. J Clin Aesthet Dermatol. 2015;8:38–42.
48. Ahmed SA, Kloezen W, Duncanson F, Zijlstra EE, de Hoog GS, Fahal AH, van de Sande WW. Madurella mycetomatis is highly susceptible to ravuconazole. PLoS Negl Trop Dis. 2014;e2942. doi: 10.1371/journal.pntd.0002942.eCollection 2014.
49. Maeda J, Nanjoh Y, Koga H, Toga T, Makimura K, Tsuboi R. In vitro fungal activity of luliconazole against Trichophyton spp. Med Mycol J. 2016;57:J1–6.
50. Shimamura T, Hasegawa N, Kubota N. Antifungal activity of luliconazole nail solution on in vitro and in vivo onychomycosis model. Med Mycol J. 2016;57:J13–8.
51. Wiederhhold NP, Fothergill AW, McCarthy DI, Tavakkol A. Luliconazole demonstrates potent in vitro activity against dermatophytes recovered from patients with onychomycosis. Antimicrob Agents Chemother. 2014;58:3553–5.
52. Khanna D, Bharti S. Luliconazole for the treatment of fungal infections: an evidence based review. Core Evid. 2014;9:113–24.
53. Machado Vila TV, Sousa Quintanilha N, Rozental S. Miltefosine is effective against *Candida albicans* and Fusarium oxysporum nail biofilms in vitro. J Med Microbiol. 2015;64:1436–49.
54. Xu Y, Miao X, Zhou B, Luo D. Combined oral terbinafine and long-pulsed 1,604-nm Nd: YAG laser treatment is more effective for onychomycosis than either treatment alone. Dermatol Surg. 2014;40:1201–7.
55. Sarifakioglu E, Şeckin D, Demirbilek M, Can F. In vitro antifungal susceptibility patterns of dermatophyte strains causing tinea unguium. Clin Exp Dermatol. 2007;32:675–9.

Chapter 23
Myths in Treating Onychomycosis

Tracey C. Vlahovic and Cara L. Dawes

Multiple times per week in a physician's practice, a practitioner will encounter a patient who asks questions regarding how onychomycosis developed in the nails and/or discusses a home remedy found on the internet that is supposed to clear onychomycosis. Any nail specialist, whether dermatologist or podiatric physician, can name a litany of the possibly logical and illogical "cures" that are displayed with a simple internet search. When faced with a patient who has tried these home remedies and has not seen the result they wanted, it is best not to judge or make light of what they have used, but instead give them the facts as to what is the possible source of the fungal infection and why common household remedies have or haven't worked.

Toenail Fungus Is Rare, So Only Those Who Don't Take Care of Their Feet Develop Onychomycosis

Since dermatophytes are ubiquitous in the environment, mycotic nail disease is the most common nail pathology worldwide reaching all cultures and ethnicities. Onychomycosis is increasing, accounting for up to 90 % of toenail and at least 50 % of fingernail infections [1]. Onychomycosis occurs in 10 % of the general population, 20 % of individuals 60 years and older, and 50 % of individuals over 70 years [2]. That said, it's not just the patient being exposed to the dermatophyte in the environment, it's also a combination of patient health and genetic predisposition to

T.C. Vlahovic, DPM, FFPM RCPS (Glasg) (✉)
Department of Podiatric Medicine, Temple University School of Podiatric Medicine, 148 N 8th Street, Philadelphia, 19107 PA, USA
e-mail: traceyv@temple.edu

C.L. Dawes, DPM
Department of Podiatry, Chestnut Hill Hospital, Philadelphia, PA, USA
e-mail: caradawesdpm@gmail.com

A. Tosti et al. (eds.), *Onychomycosis*, DOI 10.1007/978-3-319-44853-4_23

create the perfect situation for fungus to take hold. Peripheral vascular disease, immunologic disorders, and diabetes mellitus correlate with increased prevalence in older adults. The risk of onychomycosis is 1.9–2.8 times higher in persons with diabetes mellitus, and in patients with HIV infection, prevalence rates range from 15 to 40 % [2]. Other predisposing factors include older age, sex (male > female), genetic predisposition, tinea pedis (interdigital or moccasin types), peripheral arterial disease, smoking, nail trauma, inappropriate nail hygiene, and family background of onychomycosis and hyperhidrosis [2].

Adult patients constitute the bulk of those seeking treatment, but there are increasing numbers of pediatric cases, possibly due to increasing childhood obesity and pediatric diabetes. With prevalence ranging from 0 to 2.6 % worldwide, pediatric onychomycosis is relatively rare compared to adults, but still one of the most common nail disorders in children [3]. Ultimately, it is a multifactorial disease that is not solely caused by poor hygiene or poor choices of shoe gear.

Home Remedies and Over-the-Counter Products in the Foot Care Aisle Are Surefire Cures

The practitioner is often faced with hearing the following "cures" for onychomycosis on a daily basis: Listerine, Vicks VapoRub, oil of oregano, apple cider vinegar, bleach, and tea tree oil, to name a few. Patients are inundated with various remedies in the foot care aisle in their local pharmacy promising a clear nail in a small amount of time.

Apple cider vinegar (ACV) is touted as a cure all tonic for many different ailments and has websites dedicated to its properties. It is generally inexpensive and easy to obtain. Patients are bombarded with faceless, picture-less "my toenails look better!" testimonials that claim the anonymous person's nail disease was cured. What is in apple cider vinegar? Maleic acid, acetic acid, pectin, beta carotene, acetoin, methanol, alanine, ethanol, ethyl acetate, lactic acid, methanol, glycerol, and tartaric acid, in addition to mineral salts, phosphorus, potassium, chloride, sodium, and other minerals [4, 5]. It's the maleic acid that purportedly has the properties of being both bactericidal and fungicidal. Some have theorized that acetate can inhibit lanosterol demethylase which means it would impact ergosterol production in a fungal cell; others have felt that acetic acid is permeable to the cell membrane and the presence of it is toxic to the cell [6, 7].

There have been no clinical trials showing that it creates a mycological or clinical cure for onychomycosis. The closest study to dissect ACV's antifungal properties was in the Journal of Prosthodontics where the authors studied ACV for denture stomatitis which is usually caused by *Candida albicans* [4]. This study showed the MIC (minimum inhibitory concentration) of ACV versus the common antifungal for *Candida*: nystatin, but more importantly, it showed the microbial death curve. The microbial death curve is a more dynamic measure, as it allows "quantitative analysis of the fungicidal activity and of the time required until microbial death" [4], ultimately showing the behavior of antifungal agent in the presence of the organism. In this study, the kinetics of antifungal activity of ACV varied at all concentrations and time intervals from nystatin and control. All groups (ACV and nystatin) showed fungistatic activity when tested at MIC and MIC × 2, between 0 and 180 min. When tested at MIC × 4, ACV exhibited fungistatic activity only between 0 and 30 min; however after 30 min, it began to exhibit fungicidal activity. So, ultimately, for *Candida albicans*, ACV concentration and time exposed to the organism will affect whether it acts as a funstistatic agent or fungicidal agent.

When translating this to clinical practice, there are no MIC data or microbial death curves on ACV's effect on *T. rubrum* or *T. mentagrophytes*, the most common dermatophytes seen in toenail onychomycosis. Although it seems that ACV does exhibit antifungal behavior in vitro, we can't make that direct connection in vivo to onychomycosis or determine the concentration/time exposed needed to have a fungicidal effect. More studies are needed to determine what, if any, true effect can be had on fungal toenails. At this stage, it remains a folk remedy with widely varying results.

Another folk remedy that is both readily found on the Internet and recommended by physicians, Vicks VapoRub (Proctor and Gamble), an over-the-counter mentholated ointment, has been described as a treatment for onychomycosis. Many physicians feel there is a cost benefit of using an easily attainable product that has no side effects, but are unaware of the research on this product.

The components of Vicks VapoRub are thymol, menthol, camphor, and oil of *Eucalyptus* which seem to be broad-spectrum anti-infectives that have shown activity in vitro against *Candida*, *Aspergillus*, and some dermatophytes [8]. Some data has been generated about its use for toenail onychomycosis in vivo.

The first clinical trial completed using Vicks VapoRub on mycotic nails is a pilot study that was performed by a Family Medicine Group [8]. Eighteen subjects who had nail disease completed the 48-week study. There are some positive aspects of this study, but it did not follow all of the protocols that are normally done for topical antifungal studies. Unlike phase 3 clinical trials for toenail onychomycosis, this study did not exclusively enroll patients who cultured dermatophytes like *T. rubrum* or *T. mentagrophytes* and did not limit the percent of affected nail to 50 or 60 %. Instead, they allowed patients who cultured organisms like "fungal elements," *Cryptococcus*, *Candida*, *Penicillium*, and *Fusarium* and allowed up to 100 % of the nail affected visually. Of the 18 patients, only nine subjects cultured either *T. rubrum* or *T. mentagrophytes*.

Their results were the following: five of the 18 (27.8 %) had a mycological and clinical cure, and ten (55.6 %) had "partial clearance." But let's dissect this further; if we were to look at the nine subjects who cultured the most common dermatophytes causing onychomycosis, those who had *T. rubrum* fared the worst: five had partial clearance (at times only a 10 % change in the nail appearing clearer at week 48) and one had no change at all. *T. mentagrophytes* infected toenails did the best with all three subjects going onto a complete cure, but a complete cure was not defined as 0 % surface area affected—these patients still had 5 % or more of the nail visually affected at 48 weeks. Of the other organisms involved, both subjects who had *Candida parapsilosis* went onto a complete cure, but *Penicillium* species and *Candida albicans* (one subject each) had no change.

Ten of the 18 subjects had greater than 60 % nail affected at the beginning of the study—with some having 89 % or 100 % affected nails. This is highly unusual for a toenail clinical trial and certainly can be argued that a 48-week treatment period isn't long enough to manage a nail that is totally dystrophic. Adding a modality such as nail debridement could be synergistic for a topical study that enrolls nails as involved as these.

While this study is a positive start in supporting or shattering the use of a mentholated ointment for mycotic nails, it does not convince one to recommend it to patients in the office. A study that controls percent nail involvement, nail thickness, nail debridement, organisms cultured, and product use (some patients used it daily; some only three to five times per week) while having a vehicle arm and a larger sample size would create a more convincing evidence-based protocol. Time will tell if this ointment truly can eradicate fungus, or by virtue of its ointment properties, simply create a more hydrated nail unit which gives the appearance of a healthier nail.

Another readily available over-the-counter product, tea tree oil (TTO) is an essential oil derived from the leaves of *Melaleuca alternifolia* that has been described as anti-inflammatory, antibacterial, and antifungal [9]. However, it also has potential to cause skin irritation and allergic contact dermatitis [9].

When creating a topical antifungal product, one must consider the size of the particle being engineered to go through the pores of the nail plate, as well as lipophilic and hydrophilic properties of the molecule. In one study, TTO was placed in either a nanoemulsion or nanocapsule formulation that, in theory, could better penetrate the nail unit. This controlled in vitro study combined a culture of *T. rubrum*, nail powder (from healthy nails), and either formulation of the TTO. Given that nail hydration improves the penetration through the nail plate of poorly water soluble drugs, an aqueous solution would hydrate the nail keratin and possibly cause the pores to increase in size [10, 11]. Ultimately, the nanocapsule TTO had the most antifungal activity, possibly due to its being an aqueous suspension with a small particle size.

The previous study was completed in a lab and did not use human subjects. In a double-blind, randomized, controlled study comparing topical use of clotrimazole 1 % solution and TTO 100 %, subjects used either product twice daily for 6 months [12]. One hundred sixteen distal subungual onychomycosis patients who either tested culture positive for *T. rubrum* or *T. mentagrophytes* were enrolled. After 6 months, results were expressed as "culture cure" (clotrimazole = 10 %, TTO = 18 %), and clinical assessment (partial or complete cure) was clotrimazole 61 % and TTO 60 %. Adverse events which included erythema and irritation occurred more in the TTO group than the clotrimazole group. Compared to phase 3 clinical trials for onychomycosis, this is a short study that used clotrimazole as a "control." Clotrimazole solution is not an FDA-approved topical for onychomycosis and has been shown to be mildly beneficial in limited studies on nails. A more convincing protocol design would have been to incorporate a vehicle arm compared with the

TTO solution for 48 weeks. Again, these are interesting and mildly positive results, but not enough evidence to create a paradigm shift in a practice.

Remaining products that a patient would find in the pharmacy foot care aisle or in their physician's office include topicals that take their FDA approval for dermatophyte infections to the limit. Many of them show a fungally infected nail on the package, but if one reads the fine print, it will be shown that the product is indicated for the "skin around the nail" and are FDA approved for "fungal infections" or "tinea pedis." None of the products are FDA approved for the treatment of mycotic toenails. These include formulations containing undecylenic acid, clotrimazole, tolnaftate, and various antiseptics like polyhexamethylene biguanide (PHMB). In conclusion, even though the price may be reasonable and the packaging convincing, buyers should be aware that all of these products are based on creative wordsmithing, visual graphic packaging, and small data sets.

Removing a Toenail Will Kill the Fungal Infection

For a singularly painful or thickened nail, some patients may opt for total nail removal of the nail plate. Simple total avulsion of the nail itself is not curative for a mycotic nail; as the procedure has not addressed the basis of infection. Combining nail avulsion and topical antifungals has been described as the preferred treatment plan. Total nail avulsion with the use of a topical azole cream applied twice daily to the exposed nail bed resulted in a high dropout rate. All patients with total dystrophic onychomycosis failed, and only 56 % patients (15/27) were cured with this approach [13], suggesting that the procedure should not be generally recommended for the treatment of onychomycosis.

Toenail Fungus Will Go Away on Its Own

While patients seek treatment due to the cosmetic appearance of their nail, it is important the practitioner educate the patient that this is an infection. This is a medical condition that is a dermatophyte invasion of the nail bed which subsequently causes changes in both the nail bed and nail plate. Mycotic toenails are a reservoir for dermatophytes; which is why the dry skin that doesn't respond to moisturizers that patients complain about is not truly xerosis. It is tinea pedis, most likely caused by the same dermatophyte invading the nail. And vice versa, tinea pedis in the interdigital or plantar areas of the foot also acts as a reservoir for the nail [14]. Treating one of the two conditions will only lead to frustration and a suboptimal result. The skin and nail should both be treated to achieve the goals of antifungal therapy (mycological cure and visual improvement).

Within the nail itself, the infection has the potential to start distally at the hyponychium and stay in that area for months or years, or ultimately progress proximally, creating a more visually involved nail. Also, surrounding nails may become infected over time. While this slow (or in some cases medium-paced) progression hasn't been documented in a neat and predictable timeline, it has certainly been observed by patients and practitioners alike. That said, mycotic toenails will not resolve on their own without intervention. This is not a self-limiting condition.

Oral Antifungals Will "Wreck" My Liver

A common misconception among general practitioners, some specialists, and patients is the oral antifungals are designed to cause liver disease almost immediately upon ingestion and should categorically be avoided. These agents, oral terbinafine, itraconazole, and fluconazole, have been the subject of many studies to determine safety and efficacy. Of these, terbinafine and itraconazole are FDA approved for the treatment of toenail onychomycosis. Prior to placing a patient on one of these medications, it is imperative to determine the nail disease is truly a fungal infection and not one of the many differential diagnoses. Second, a thorough history and physical with pertinent blood work should be done before the first dose is taken. As with any medication, patient selection is key. Finally, the safety of these medications was elegantly dissected in a meta-analysis that involved 122 studies that enrolled 20,000 patients. The pooled risks of treatment discontinuation result from adverse reactions for continuous therapy of terbinafine (250 mg/day, 3.44 %), itraconazole (100 mg/day, 4.21 %), pulsed terbinafine (2.09 %), pulsed itraconazole (2.58 %), and intermittent fluconazole (150 mg/week, 1.98 %) [15]. The risk of liver injury requiring termination of the medication ranged from 0.11 % (continuous itraconazole) to 1.22 % (continuous fluconazole). The risk of liver function values elevating asymptomatically and not requiring treatment or discontinuation of therapy was less than 2 % for all regimens evaluated. Therefore, in an immucompetent population, the risk of adverse events when taking these oral antifungal medications is low. Of course, oral antifungal medications aren't for every patient, but the sustaining myth that liver damage is imminent in a healthy population should be reexamined by those who have been perpetuating that belief for years.

Toenail Fungus Can't Be Cured: Topicals and Orals Don't Work

"Cure" is a challenging word, as it denotes absolute finality. Treating mycotic nails is not like treating a superficial skin infection with an antibiotic. As anyone who has treated or developed mycotic toenails understands, it has the potential to recur for various reasons. One must be diligent about not only in managing this clinical entity pharmacologically but also managing the environment (socks, shoes, shared shower spaces) and educating the patient that their predisposition (genetic or medical condition) may cause them to revisit this diagnosis in the future [16]. Concomitant tinea pedis should be treated along with the nail. Patients should be educated on the first signs of either nail disease or skin involvement to seek treatment.

It has been well documented the effectiveness of both the oral and topical antifungal medications in the treatment of this infection (Chapters 19, 20). Again, these agents will assist the nails to achieve a mycological and visual cure, but the environment must be considered and managed in order to obtain a longer state of clear nail (and skin).

Patient expectations must be managed. Often, the nails have been mycotic for years which can cause permanent nail changes. Once a mycological cure has been achieved, the nails may always have some degree of dystrophy which visually will appear disappointing. Also, if the nails are affected by patient biomechanics (i.e., a hammertoe on a lesser digit), the nails may always appear onychauxic due to the chronic repetitive trauma those nails are subject to. Patient education is key that nails are subject to the environment and forces around them and are in flux.

References

1. Ghannoum MA, Hajjeh RA, Scher R, et al. A large-scale North American study of fungal isolates from nails: the frequency of onychomycosis, fungal distribution, and antifungal susceptibility patterns. J Am Acad Dermatol. 2000;43:641–8.
2. Westerberg DP, Yoyack MJ. Onychomycosis: current trends in diagnosis and treatment. Am Fam Physician. 2013;88(11):762–70.
3. Gupta AK, Skinner AR, Baran R. Onychomycosis in children: an overview. J Drugs Dermatol. 2003;2:31–4.
4. Mota AC et al. Antifungal activity of apple cider vinegar on candida species involved in denture stomatitis. J Prosthodont. 2015;24(4):296–302.
5. Heikefelt C. Chemical and sensory analyses of juice, cider and vinegar produced from different apple cultivars. Alnarp: Swedish University of Agricultural Sciences, Faculty of Landscape Planning, Horticulture and Agricultural Sciences, Department of Plant Breeding and Biotechnology; 2011.
6. Arneborg N, Jespersen L, Jakobsen M. Individual cells of *Saccharomyces cerevisiae* and Zygosaccharomyces bailii exhibit different short-term intracellular pH responses to acetic acid. Arch Microbiol. 2000;174:125–8.
7. Guldfeldt L, Arneborg U. Measurement of the effects of acetic acid and extracellular pH on intracellular pH of nonfermenting, individual *Saccharomyces cerevisiae* cells by fluorescence microscopy. Appl Environ Microbiol. 1998;64:530–4.
8. Derby R, Rohal P, Jackson C, et al. Treatment of onychomycosis using mentholated ointment. J Am Board Fam Med. 2011;24:69–74.
9. Flores FC, de Lima JA, Ribeiro RF, Alves SH, Rolim CM, Beck RC, da Silva CB. Antifungal activity of nanocapsule suspensions containing tea tree oil on the growth of Trichophyton rubrum. Mycopathologia. 2013;175(3–4):281–6.
10. Gunt H, Kasting GB. Effect of hydration on the permeation of ketoconazole through human nail plate in vitro. Eur J Pharm Sci. 2007;32:254–60.
11. Murdan S. Drug delivery to the nail following topical application. Int J Pharm. 2002;236: 1–26.

12. Buck DS, Nidorf DM, Addino JG. Comparison of two topical preparations for the treatment of onychomycosis: melaleuca alternifolia (tea tree) oil and clotrimazole. J Fam Pract. 1994; 38(6):601–5.
13. Grover C, Bansal S, Nanda S, et al. Combination of surgical avulsion and topical therapy for single nail onychomycosis: a randomized controlled trial. Br J Dermatol. 2007;157(2):364–8.
14. Vlahovic TC, Joseph WS, Scher RK, Tosti A, Plasencia J, Pariser DM, Markinson BC. Diagnosis and management of onychomycosis: perspectives from a joint podiatry-dermatology roundtable. J Am Podiatr Med Assoc. 2016;106(2):155–62.
15. Chang CH, Young-Xu Y, Kurth T, Orav JE, Chan AK. The safety of oral antifungal treatments for superficial dermatophytosis and onychomycosis: a meta-analysis. Am J Med. 2007;120: 791–8. (B)
16. Gupta AK, Paquet M. Improved efficacy in onychomycosis therapy. Clin Dermatol. 2013;31:555–63.

Index

A. Tosti et al. (eds.), *Onychomycosis*, DOI 10.1007/978-3-319-44853-4

O

MIX
Papier aus verantwortungsvollen Quellen
Paper from responsible sources
FSC® C105338

If you have any concerns about our products,
you can contact us on
ProductSafety@springernature.com

In case Publisher is established outside the EU,
the EU authorized representative is:
Springer Nature Customer Service Center GmbH
Europaplatz 3, 69115 Heidelberg, Germany

Printed by Libri Plureos GmbH
in Hamburg, Germany